Mental Health Social Work in Context

There has been a re-energising of interest in social work's role in mental health services in recent years and mental health is now a core part of all qualifying social work students' training.

Grounded in the social models of mental health particularly relevant to qualifying social workers, but also familiarising students with social aspects of medical perspectives, this core text helps to prepare students for practice and to develop their knowledge around:

- promoting the social inclusion of people with mental health problems;

- the changing context of multidisciplinary mental health services;

- an integrated evidence base for practice;

- working with people with mental health problems across the life course.

Mental Health Social Work in Context is an essential textbook for all social work students taking undergraduate and postgraduate qualifying degrees in social work, and will also be invaluable for practitioners undertaking post-qualifying awards in mental health social work.

Nick Gould is Professor of Social Work at the University of Bath, recognised internationally for his writing and research, and has held visiting appointments in Australia and Hong Kong. Since qualifying as a social worker over thirty years ago, he has combined an academic career with maintaining direct involvement in front-line practice, including serving for many years as a member of the Mental Health Review Tribunal. From 2003–6 he was the National Institute for Mental Health England's Fellow in Social Care Research and Practice.

Student Social Work

This exciting new textbook series is ideal for all students studying to be qualified social workers, whether at undergraduate or masters level. Covering key elements of the social work curriculum, the books are accessible, interactive and thought-provoking.

New titles

Human Growth and Development
An introduction for social workers
John Sudbery

Social Work and Social Policy
An introduction
Jonathan Dickens

Social Work Placements
Mark Doel

Forthcoming titles

Integrating Social Work Theory and Practice
Pam Green Lister

Social Work
A reader
Vivienne E. Cree

Building Relationships and Communicating with Young Children
A practical guide
Karen Winter

Mental Health Social Work in Context

Nick Gould

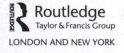

Routledge
Taylor & Francis Group

LONDON AND NEW YORK

First published 2010
by Routledge
2 Park Square, Milton Park, Abingdon, Oxon OX14 4RN

Simultaneously published in the USA and Canada
by Routledge
270 Madison Avenue, New York, NY 10016

Reprinted 2011

Routledge is an imprint of the Taylor & Francis Group, an informa business

© 2010 Nick Gould

Typeset in Times New Roman by
Keystroke, Tettenhall, Wolverhampton

Printed and bound in Great Britain by
TJ International Ltd, Padstow, Cornwall

British Library Cataloguing in Publication Data
A catalogue record for this book is available from the British Library

Library of Congress Cataloging-in-Publication Data
 Gould, Nick.
 Mental health social work in context / Nick Gould.
   p. cm.
 Includes bibliographical references.
 1. Psychiatric social work. I. Title.
 HV689.G67 2010
 362.2'0425—dc22   2009020721

ISBN10: 0–415–45201–5 (hbk)
ISBN10: 0–415–45203–1 (pbk)
ISBN10: 0–203–86541–3 (ebk)

ISBN13: 978–0–415–45201–4 (hbk)
ISBN13: 978–0–415–45203–8 (pbk)
ISBN13: 978–0–203–86541–5 (ebk)

To Hilary

Contents

Contents

Activities

Introduction

> Social work and social workers are important. Social work makes an important contribution to mental health services and is a crucial component in their development. . . . However, like any other profession, social workers cannot afford to rest on their laurels and stand still.
>
> (Department of Health 2007b: 117)

This book has been written in the spirit of the message conveyed by this quotation from a fairly recent official report about the development of the mental health workforce. It is premised on a conviction that social work makes a vital contribution to services for people with mental health problems, but it has been written with an awareness that in many parts of the profession there are significant anxieties about the capacity of social work to sustain its identity and distinct contribution in the context of rapidly changing contexts of practice. There are particular concerns about the integration of health and social care services and the location of social work within multidisciplinary structures where social work is the minority player, and is heavily outnumbered by medical and ancillary professionals. Consequently, one purpose in writing this book was to delineate the changing context of practice, describing the policy environment that is shaping these changes, the implications for interventions to support people with mental health problems, and in particular the relevance of all this for the role of the social worker.

The primary intended readership for this book is students who are studying for an undergraduate or Masters degree that qualifies them to be a professional social worker. The book will have particular relevance for those who intend to practise after qualification in a mental health setting. However, mental health is part of the generic professional curriculum for all qualifying social workers, and consequently this book has relevance for all students of social work. Indeed, this reflects the evidence that users of all areas of social care services, including children's as well as adult services, experience disproportionate levels of mental health problems. To be effective in any setting, social workers need to have some knowledge of the main forms of mental disorder, their presentation and the kinds of intervention that are shown by evidence to be effective.

This book is intended to reflect social perspectives drawn from the social and policy sciences, as well as incorporating some knowledge from clinical psychiatry. It consciously attempts not to proselytise for something often referred to as 'the social model' because of the reductionist implications of this phrase and its inference that there is a unitary model that can be contrasted with something equally unproblematically understood as 'the medical model'. This book steers a middle course that acknowledges the problematic and contested nature of medical psychiatry, and advocates for psychological and social interventions where they have been demonstrated to be beneficial, but at the same time acknowledges that there are forms of pharmacological and other medical interventions that offer some respite for some people from mental distress. It also recognises that an important source of 'evidence' in relation to best practice is the perspective offered by people who use services themselves, the 'experts by experience'. All this may be imperfect and untidy but offers the best options we have at present. I accept that the consequence of adopting this position is that some readers will find the content too uncritical of psychiatry as a disciplinary practice, while others will feel it accommodates too much to social perspectives! However, if social workers are to promote their position within integrated mental health services they need to be able to articulate how their own social perspectives relate to (and sometimes critique and challenge) mainstream psychiatric practice.

For the same reasons, social workers need to have a broad familiarity with the main systems of classification of mental disorders used in psychiatry. There are two classification systems used in the context of UK mental health services. The 'ICD-10 classification of mental and behavioural disorders: clinical descriptions and diagnostic guidelines' is the fifth chapter of the World Health Organization's tenth revision of the *International Classification of Diseases and Health Related Problems* (World Health Organization 1992). This guideline (hereafter referred to as *ICD-10*) provides clinical descriptions, diagnostic criteria, and criteria for research for mental health and behavioural disorders and is in common use internationally. In 1994 the American Psychiatric Association produced an alternative classification system, the *Diagnostic and Statistical Manual of Mental Disorders*, also widely adopted, currently in its fourth revision and usually referred to as *DSM-IV* (American Psychiatric Association 1994). Clinicians may have a preference for one classification system over the other, but they are broadly complementary and are often used interchangeably by psychiatrists. There are numerous critiques of the validity of categorising mental disorder, not least whether some or all mental states exist on continua of experience rather than being fixed categories or traits (Goldberg and Huxley 1992; Bentall 2003). The purpose of referring to these major diagnostic systems in subsequent chapters of this book is not to reproduce uncritically a medical perspective, but to help social workers make an informed contribution to interdisciplinary practice.

Chapter 1 engages further with the debates about the dominance of psychiatry as a form of discourse, and sets out some of the models of mental disorder that influence practice and service development, including the so-called medical, social and psychosocial models. It also reviews emergent social perspectives that are influencing practice such as social capital theory, disability theory and the recovery model and how they are being synthesised within the 'new social models'. Chapter 2 continues the examination of social perspectives and in particular identifies some of the dimensions on which people with mental health problems experience disadvantage and multiple forms of social exclusion, including employment, housing, income and physical health. Implications for social work practice of these forms of social disadvantage are considered, including the need to sustain forms of practice that are anti-discriminatory and anti-oppressive in addressing race and ethnicity, gender and sexual orientation.

Chapter 3 brings the focus to bear on the development of the social work role in the context of the transition from institutional to community-based care. There have been some continuities in the role of the social worker, not least as a mediator between the social context within which the service user experiences their mental distress and the individualistic focus of the 'medical gaze'. The chapter also considers the significance of changing models of service delivery including service integration, care management and the personalisation agenda, and their impacts on the role of the social worker. Implications of these contextual changes are considered for the maintenance of values-based practice, and the development of key skills for mental health social work.

Chapters 4, 5 and 6 outline the main mental health issues relating to stages of the life course. In Chapter 4 the common mental health problems of children and young people are described including behavioural, developmental and emotional disorders, and relevant interventions and their justifications are discussed. There is also increasing recognition that concerns for the welfare of children can arise where their parents have mental health problems, and the complexities of engaging with these parents is also examined. This need to consider the whole family raises the problem of coordinating services between children's and adult services. Chapter 5 considers some of the mental health problems that usually have their onset in adulthood, looking particularly at mood disorders such as depression, bipolar disorder, anxiety and phobias. The signs of these problems are described and evidence-based interventions to address them are considered, particularly those which can be delivered by social workers. Chapter 6 continues the theme of mental health problems in adulthood, addressing the psychoses – particularly schizophrenia – and also considering the personality disorders.

Discussion of the social work role in relation to mental health often overlooks the fact that the largest number of service users receiving support because of mental health related problems will be older people with age-related conditions. Chapter 7 looks at mental health social work with older people including the nature of ageism and negative stereotypes of older people and their mental health. The chapter considers types and signs of dementia, the support needs of carers, the influence of Tom Kitwood's model of person-centred care and the scope for social work contributions to dementia care. The consideration of mental health in older age tends to be dominated by dementia and it is possible for practitioners to overlook the more commonly occurring incidence of depression. This is discussed, as well as the needs of people who have mental health issues that continue from earlier stages of their adult life.

Chapter 8 addresses the sometimes controversial area of the risks that can be presented by people experiencing mental health problems. This discussion is set in the context of sociological theorising about the nature of the 'risk society'; this helps to understand some of the dynamics behind the processes that amplify and exaggerate the risk to the public presented by people with a mental health problem. At the same time, practitioners need to be able to identify those situations where there are elevated levels of risk; usually this is risk to self, but some mental health conditions and situational factors are associated with increased risk to others. The role of the social worker in relation to statutory powers and the use of compulsion are reviewed, and consideration is given to the specialist role played by social work in secure settings.

Finally, Chapter 9 presents an overview of current and future challenges for social work practice with people who have mental health problems. Some of this is being addressed more broadly by policy-makers in relation to a wide spectrum of professionals who practise within rapidly changing mental health services, and the implications for social work of this 'new ways of working' programme are considered along with the relevance to social work of attempts to define generic core competencies in mental health practice, particularly the 'Ten Essential Shared Capabilities'. This leads on to consideration of the place of social work within the continuing evolution of specialist – so-called 'functional' – teams, and the advantages and disadvantages of expecting professionals in multidisciplinary teams to demonstrate generic, core capabilities. The chapter also provides an overview of other emergent issues for mental health social work including the development of leadership capacity, the challenges of working across organisational boundaries, the possible impact of the personalisation agenda, the need to develop research capacity, and future engagement in mental health policy development.

This book draws on my involvement of over more than three decades in social work and mental health services. There are too many people to mention individually, including many service users, whose influence and inspiration have kept my interest and commitment in this area of work alive. However, there are some groups of people to whom I am especially indebted. I have been very fortunate that for many years my place of employment has been the University of Bath, and colleagues within the Department of Social and Policy Sciences are a constant source of support and stimulation. From 2003 until 2006 I held a fellowship awarded by the National Institute for Mental Health England and Social Care Institute for Excellence; this was an invaluable opportunity to focus my research and writing around the development of evidence-based practice in mental health, as well as providing a platform for continuing collaboration with national health and social care agencies on the development of guidelines for good practice. The fellowship was also an opportunity to work with an inspirational alliance of service users, professionals and academics, the Social Perspectives Network. Not least, for many years I have been a member of the Mental Health Review Tribunal, which has sustained my involvement in forensic aspects of mental health work and provided the opportunity to work alongside skilled and dedicated legal and medical colleagues.

The lifestyle of an academic is not easy for loved ones; the research and writing processes seem to require periods of self-absorption, remoteness and downright selfishness. My wife, Hilary, as well as being an inspiration through her own dedication to working with children and families, has always encouraged and supported me to believe that goals could be achieved, including bringing this book to fruition. She played a major part in persuading me that this might be a point in my career to write for a student readership, rather than always addressing the academic and research communities. Our children, Miles and Alice, have also been indulgent of my pre-occupations and are a constant source of humour and good questions. My step-daughters, Sarah and Jo, are both active in areas of work addressed by this book, and give me encouragement that there are younger people ready to become involved in working with people who experience mental distress.

My mother, the late Jean Gould, has often been in my mind as I wrote this book. She sometimes had fragile mental health, an outcome of a childhood dominated by the financial insecurity of a household where her father had lost his pit job in the 1926 miners' strike and who experienced his physical health subsequently being destroyed by hard manual labouring jobs. Perhaps the most formative moment in my own upbringing was one day in a school holiday when my mother took me on a guided tour of the University of Oxford. She lived to see that I would become a postgraduate student at the same university, but not that my career would centre on social aspects of mental health and themes prefigured in her own early life. My father, Harry ('Hal') Gould, has seen this and his lifelong influences on me as a teacher, philosopher, raconteur and flamenco guitarist are beyond any words I have to thank him. Despite these many acknowledgements and thanks, it is important to emphasise that any errors and omissions from this book are entirely my own responsibility.

1 Perspectives on mental health

By the end of this chapter you should have an understanding of:

- The extent and cost of mental health problems in society

- The factors contributing to the transition from institutional to community-based care

- The main dimensions of the so-called 'medical model' and the controversies that surround it

- Social capital theory, disability theory, the recovery model and their relevance to mental health

- Essential characteristics of 'new social models' in mental health and some of the challenges to their adoption.

Introduction

Consider the following three scenarios:

> Brian is a man in his late seventies who was widowed five years ago and now lives alone in the rural community where he has resided all his life. He worked as a farm labourer and the care of his home and other domestic affairs were managed by his late wife, and he has no children or extended family. Neighbours contact social services to report that Brian has been wandering in the village, inappropriately clothed for the weather, and asking people what day of the week it is.

> Poppy is a lone parent who originates from Eritrea and now lives with her two teenage children in a house rented from the local authority. Twelve months ago she began complaining to the police that an unknown person was breaking into her house when she was out and moving her belongings, but the police could find no evidence to substantiate this claim. Poppy has now been referred by her GP to the local Community Mental Health Team as she was complaining to her doctor that she could not sleep, and attributed this to unidentified persons shouting abusive comments about her at night. When the team social worker visits Poppy's house she finds that windows and doors are barricaded and the whole family is sleeping in a downstairs room for protection against unknown aggressors.

> Jeremy is a man in his early twenties who has lived with his parents since dropping out of university during his first year of studies, citing as reasons for doing this that he had lost interest in his subject and that he would find a job. He has never secured employment and now spends all his time in his bedroom where he also takes his meals. Jeremy's parents report that he spends all day writing in notebooks or staring into space.

All these situations are not untypical of those that a social worker might be called on to assess, and possibly follow up, either alone or with others as part of a multidisciplinary team approach. Each situation contains ambiguities and uncertainties that could be indicative of the presence of a mental health problem, or they may be the consequence of social circumstances, or a combination of factors. It may even transpire that the person concerned does not consider that they have a problem; the difficulty may be the attitudes of those who define the person's behaviour as problematic.

Whatever the particular circumstances behind these scenarios, the thesis behind this book is that in order to practise effectively social workers need an understanding of the social factors that impact on mental health. Furthermore, because social workers increasingly practise in contexts where they work alongside members of other professions, they also need an appreciation of the various frameworks that inform their decision-making – be they medical, psychological or legal perspectives. They also need to be responsive to perspectives that are based on the philosophy that the best understandings come from those who themselves have mental health problems and use services, the 'experts by experience'.

Though it may try the patience of the reader who wishes to press on with learning about specific mental health conditions – perhaps schizophrenia or dementia – because of the contested nature of mental health, we first have to spend some time considering the wider frameworks or approaches that will shape our understanding and therefore our practice. The approach taken by this book is not, however, that mental health problems are entirely constructed by language and its meaning and context, a perspective that is sometimes described as 'social constructivism' (Burr 1995). Nor on the other hand is this book advocating biological determinism, the assumption that all mental health problems are ultimately physiological, and which consigns social workers to being the 'hand maidens' of psychiatrists. The position taken is one sometimes described by the label of 'pragmatism', not as in the lay definition that anything will do as long as it works, but in the more technical, philosophical sense that we have to work with the best evidence that we currently have – namely, that all knowledge should be considered as provisional and subject to review as mental health becomes better understood.

This pragmatic perspective is combined with critical realism, the view that mental disorder is something that has an external reality, and can be detected and measured, but that it exists within social contexts and that social workers have a responsibility to be both critical and proactive about its inequitable and discriminatory consequences. Tew seems to be expressing a similar position in an article about social perspectives and social work education:

> Rather than taking the extreme position that 'mental illness' does not exist, a social model need not rule out the possibility that some people may have greater innate vulnerabilities to particular experiences due to medical, nutritional, genetic or other factors. However, over and above any biological predisposing factors, evidence suggests that a variety of social factors may play a major role in contributing to longer-term vulnerability to breakdown or distress.
>
> (Tew 2002)

The scale of the problems

Mental ill-health, despite the stigmatisation it can produce, is everyone's business. At any point in time around 16 per cent of the population in Britain are experiencing a common mental health disorder such as depression (Beddington et al., 2008). Around 4 per cent will be living with a severe mental disorder such as schizophrenia or bipolar affective disorder. In the region of 700,000 people are experiencing dementia in the UK, which will rise to over one million by 2025 (Alzheimer's Society 2007). Although there is some variation in diagnostic rates between countries, for instance prevalence rates for depression of 4 per cent in Shanghai and 26 per cent in the United States, reflecting cultural and service differences, it is increasingly recognised that mental ill-health is a major factor in the global experience of ill-health and disability (Desjarlais et al., 1996). Measuring the so-called Global Burden of Disease in terms of Daily-Adjusted Life Years the World Health Organization (2002) found that: neuropsychiatric disorders comprised 13 per cent of the global burden of disease; neuropsychiatric disorders contribute four of the ten leading causes of disability; neuropsychiatric disorders contribute 28 per cent of years of life lived with a disability; depression accounts for over 12 per cent of years of life lived with a disability. These are twice the levels of disability caused by cancer (5.3 per cent) and higher than the level of disability caused by cardiovascular disease (10.3 per cent) (Thornicroft and Tansella 2004).

If politicians and policy-makers are still not persuaded by the magnitude of these challenges, the economic analyses of the costs of mental disorder are likely to focus their minds. A study for the European Union calculated that the total costs of mental disorders are about 3–4 per cent of Gross National Product (STAKES 1999). The indirect costs due to lack of productivity resulting from exclusion from the labour market multiply this figure even further: a study in the UK estimated that the annual cost of mental distress to the national economy was around £77 billion (Sainsbury Centre for Mental Health 2003). Without committing us to a narrowly utilitarian view of this, that is, defining something as a problem simply because it is costly for the wider economy, these figures do provide some kind of proxy of the amount of distress and disruption that are caused in the lives of individuals by mental health problems.

This chapter provides a brief historical overview of the emergence of community-based care for people with mental health problems, it reviews the arguments for and against adopting a medical perspective on the experience of mental distress, and then considers a range of perspectives that contribute to contemporary understandings of mental disorder, including the biopsychosocial model, social capital, the disability movement, recovery perspectives and, finally, a drawing together of core aspects of the 'new' social models.

From the asylum to community care

Even within the working lifetime of many current mental health social workers the dominant paradigm for the delivery of mental health care has changed dramatically. Research by Huxley et al. (2003) has shown that the mental health social work workforce is predominantly middle aged. Practitioners may well have developed their interest and expertise in mental health when the dominant mode of intervention for people with a mental health problem was in-patient treatment (often long term) in a large hospital, probably a 'county asylum' first built in the mid-nineteenth century. The publicity surrounding scandals of patient abuse (Butler and Drakeford 2005), the escalating costs of maintaining large hospitals (Scull 1977), the availability of powerful tranquilising drugs to suppress symptoms (Rose 2007), and an intellectual climate of radicalism combined in the 1960s to challenge the dominant form of in-patient care, what Foucault had likened to the segregation of lepers in the Middle Ages (Foucault 1961).

At that time 'anti-psychiatry' was in the ascendancy, a broad umbrella for a range of intellectual influences including social constructionism and labelling theory, the Palo Alto school of systems theory and, not least, R. D. Laing's beguiling cocktail of existentialism, psychedelia and (briefly) Marxist dialectic (Gould 2005). For a period in the late 1960s and early 1970s it seemed that these influences would synthesise into an irresistible defeat of the dominant medical approach to treating mental distress. In fact, apart from some exceptions such as *Psichatria Democratica* in Italy (a radical alliance of political activists and psychiatrists whose agitation led in 1978 to legislation to close all Italian public mental hospitals) (Donnelly 1992), this was no more triumphant than the student and worker protests of the same period were in overthrowing the capitalist order. As various commentators have pointed out, anti-psychiatry was more potent as a rallying point for cultural disaffection than it was as a serious response to the complexities of the lives of people who were mentally distressed (Sedgwick 1982; Miller and Rose 1986).

The closure of the county asylums and the transfer of care to services to the community has a more mundane rationale than the attention of the counter-culture. One credible perspective is that since the end of the Second World War we have seen the progressive dismantling of the workhouse system which had provided shelter for people with a range of disabilities and social problems (Fawcett and Karban 2005). From the 1960s the closure of long-stay provision for a range of service users accelerated, for a variety of fiscal, humanitarian and professional reasons already mentioned above. This process accelerated in the 1980s with health services looking to the private sector to alleviate the through-care problems of patients stuck in expensive hospital placements. Local authorities similarly were looking to non-statutory alternatives in order to meet demand for services, and all of this was against the background of a Conservative political orthodoxy that promoted the rolling back of the state and individual self-help.

These piecemeal developments were given policy coherence by the 1986 Audit Commission report *Making a Reality of Community Care* (1986), which identified the wastefulness of the system and pointed to the possibilities for coordinated non-institutional care arrangements that could potentially be delivered by adopting the US-developed model of case management. This led to the so-called Griffith report of 1988 and eventually the 1989 White Paper *Caring For People* (Department of Health 1989), which created the organisational architecture for care in the community, given statutory force by the National Health Service Community Care Act 1990. Despite continuous processes of reform of the internal structure and workings of health and social services, this legislation created the fundamental framework that still persists of a mixed economy of care, assessment of need and coordination of packages of care through care management, and an emphasis on care that is provided in the home or in smaller facilities located as close as possible to home.

The specifics of the reform of mental health care in Britain should not distract us from the fact that the same trends of decarceration from long-stay institutions has been taking place across the developed world, albeit with different speeds of transition (Thornicroft and Tansella 2004). The mental health system that has developed in Britain shares various generic features of other modern mental health systems. What Thornicroft and Tansella describe as the core features of contemporary mainstream mental health care, based on comparative international data, include the following: out-patient and ambulatory clinics, community mental health teams, a system of case management, acute in-patient care, long-term community-based residential care, and employment and occupation services. Countries with relatively high levels of resources, such as Britain, are characterised by the further, ongoing development of more specialised and differentiated services including: specialised outpatient clinics (e.g., for drug misusers or people with personality disorders), specialised or functional community mental health teams (e.g., assertive outreach teams and early intervention teams), alternatives to acute in-patient care (e.g., acute day hospitals, crisis house and home treatment teams), alternative long-stay community residential care (e.g., staffed residential care, supported accommodation and family placements) and new forms of supported employment. The specific mix of services and balance between forms of service varies between countries and between regions, depending on historical patterns of care, assessments of local need, and political decision-making about levels of funding.

Activity 1.1 Historical patterns of service delivery

Using public websites for local health and social care services, and any relevant documents you can access, identify which were the large mental hospitals for the area in which you live or work. Compare this with the pattern and location of the current statutory mental health services in your area. Do they seem to be located on the basis of current need, or on historical bases of old institutions?

This is the normative, uncritical vision of community care. Its adequacy in meeting the specific needs of people with mental health problems has been and continues to be problematic. As we shall see in more detail in later chapters of the book, community care has not avoided the creation of processes of institutionalisation of service users, the so-called 'new' long-stay patients, nor the systematic oversight of needs of marginalised social groups, particularly members of black and minority ethnic groups. Indeed, often it seems that mental health is a 'bolt on' to the bigger vision for health and social care. Policy for the National Health Service (NHS) is framed primarily in terms of treatment for physical health problems, and it is then translated into a mental health version. Later in the book we will consider the problems that continue for mental health managers and practitioners in accommodating to generic policy themes such as choice, personalisation and individualisation. The times when the mental health agenda comes to the fore and instigates policy reforms have usually been moments of crisis, often associated with moral panics about public safety. These tensions are explored in more depth at various points in this book, particularly in relation to the development of mental health law and forensic services (see Chapter 8).

Chapter 8

The remainder of this chapter provides a brief overview of important perspectives in mental health, beginning with medical models, but then with a focus on emergent social models, and concludes with an attempt to delineate the essential core elements of those models.

The medical model

There is no definitive statement of what constitutes the medical model, also sometimes referred to as the 'disease model'. It tends to be used by non-medical commentators on the approach taken within psychiatry that proceeds from an assumption that there are mental illnesses which can be described in terms of diagnostic categories, and that are more or less amenable to intervention by medical practitioners. As such, the forms of discourse which address the medical model tend to be inherently critical for its lack of consideration of psychological and, particularly, social factors implicated in mental distress. However, it is rather difficult to find clinicians or academics who uncritically sign up to the biological reductionism – the 'straw man' – that is sometimes implied by the term 'the medical model', though it may be a fairer assessment to say that mainstream approaches to psychiatry have tended to prioritise pharmacological interventions. However, as we see in later chapters, many guidelines based on 'evidence-based medicine' acknowledge that psychosocial approaches are in some circumstances as effective as drugs. A more subtle appreciation of what constitutes the medical model would be to say that it is an approach to problem-solving that is based on assessment, diagnosis, classification and expert intervention. As such, it is not conceptually so different from a number of structured mainstream approaches in social work, which might be cause of some reflection for those who use the term 'medical model' simply as a pejorative label.

There are clear indications that some psychiatrists and others believe that what they perceive as demonisation of the medical model has gone far enough, what even a social work professor has called 'a parody of a parody' (Pritchard, C. 2006: 48). Some psychiatrists and are now seeking to retrieve the medical model, typified by an editorial article in the *British Journal of Psychiatry* by Shah and Mountain (2007: 375) who proclaim that, 'The medical model is dead – long live the medical model'. They argue that the debates about the nature of psychiatry have fallen into an unhelpful polarisation that reflects the traditional Descartian opposition between mind and body:

> Biological psychiatry is assumed to be mechanistic and reductionist, exclusively concerned with neuroimaging, genetics and medication. Psychosocial psychiatry, championed as being empowering, humane and holistic, is regarded as the antithesis and aligns itself to models such as Engel's [see 'The Biopsychosocial Model' below for a discussion of Engel](1977).
>
> (Shah and Mountain 2007: 375)

Shah and Mountain argue that biological, social and psychological experiences are all translated into changes in brain structure and function. They cite evidence in relation to the effects of child sexual abuse, differences in personality traits, and the effects of psychological and pharmacological treatments, to the effect that they all produce physiological changes at the level of discrete brain systems. They claim on the basis of this that it is not tenable to maintain that the mind and the body are separate entities: we have a cultural reluctance to accept that anything as sanctified and rarefied as 'the mind' could be explained in terms of our biological make-up. Shah and Mountain go on to assert that psychiatrists should reassert the contribution of the medical model in terms of the expertise of doctors:

> We believe that we need a simple definition of the medical model, which incorporates medicine's fundamental ideals, to facilitate clarity and precision, without denying its shortcomings. We propose that the 'medical model' is a process whereby, informed by the best available evidence, doctors advise on, coordinate or deliver interventions for health improvement. It can be summarily stated as 'does it work?'
>
> (Shah and Mountain 2007: 375)

It will be noted that this redefinition of the medical model is primarily based on a restatement of the traditional status of the doctor, though there is also an additional claim for the authority of evidence-based medicine on the grounds that psychiatrists should offer treatments on the basis of whether they work, rather than any ideological allegiances to schools of thought. This of course begs the questions as to who defines what 'works' means in this context, and who will determine how it is measured? For these reasons this particular retrieval of the medical model is unlikely to be very persuasive to upholders of social perspectives whether they are practitioners from other disciplines or advocates for service user empowerment.

A more subtle case for a medical model that bears consideration was put forward some years ago by the late Anthony Clare who, before his rise to prominence as a 'celebrity psychiatrist', wrote a book which has been a rallying point for a pluralistic approach to mental health, *Psychiatry in Dissent* (1977). Clare identifies four orientations to mental illness: the 'organic orientation' which would equate with a deterministic biological view that mental disorder is caused by a physiological abnormality, even if the nature of that physical basis has not yet been discovered; the 'psychotherapeutic orientation' that claims that mental distress is the product of psychological conflicts within the inner world of the patient; the 'sociotherapeutic approach' that emphasises the social and environmental causes of mental problems; and the fourth orientation which Clare describes as the 'medical model' but is in fact derived from a combination of the previous three perspectives:

> The medical model, in short, takes into account not merely the symptom, syndrome or disease, but the person who suffers, his personal and social situation, his biological, psychological and social status. The medical model, as applied to psychiatry, embodies the basic principle that every illness is the product of two factors – of environment working on the organism.
>
> (Clare 1977: 70)

Clare's formulation of the medical model has been described as a 'form of inclusive compromise' (Pilgrim 2002) or a 'portmanteau model' (Baruch and Treacher 1978). His attempt at a consensus position is still too medicalised for some socially orientated commentators as he still wishes to retain the concept of illness, and the basic 'heuristic' (approach to problem-solving) of medicine that involves assessment, diagnosis and treatment by an expert. Nevertheless, Clare's writing has been influential and has much in common with the biopsychosocial model.

The biopsychosocial model

The biopsychosocial model is sometimes contrasted with the 'biomedical model', the latter being an alternative term for the medical model. The intellectual basis of the biopsychosocial model is usually taken to be general systems theory, which was developed within the biological sciences and is associated with the work of the biologists Paul Weiss and Ludwig von Bertalanffy. The main claims of general systems theory are three-fold: that mental states occur within individuals who are members of a whole system; the whole system is both sub-personal, comprising physical entities such as the nervous system, and supra-personal, made up of a psychosocial context which exists like the layers of the onion in increasing complexity as we look outwards from the individual – dyad, family, community, culture, society and biosphere. An implication of this conceptual framework is that phenomena appearing at the individual level can only be explained by reference to the outer levels of the system, so avoiding reductionism. In psychiatry the implications of general systems theory and the biopsychosocial model were elaborated primarily by Meyer (collected works published posthumously, 1952) in the first part of the twentieth century, and then by Engel (1980). They argue that on the basis of general systems theory, any attempt to explain mental disorder solely by reference to the sub-personal, that is, physiological, system will inevitably be reductionist and scientifically incomplete: explanations have to include reference to the psychological and societal levels of the system, hence the 'biopsychosocial model'.

Some time has been taken to set out these intellectual antecedents because often the label of the 'biopsychosocial model' is used as a rather lazy shortcut to describe a pragmatic approach to understanding mental disorder that reduces to mixing in a bit of everything. This tends to underplay both the coherence of the model and the specific influences it has had, particularly on British theory and practice. In an important paper reviewing the historical role of the biopsychosocial model, Pilgrim (2002) argues that the biopsychosocial model, for a period of the 1970s and 1980s, established something approaching an orthodoxy based on British centres of excellence in psychiatry such as the Maudsley hospital. It also influenced an enduring research legacy which spanned psychiatry and the social sciences:

> As a further indication of the BPS model reaching the status of a temporary orthodoxy, at least in London, it came to gain the support of collaborating psychiatric social workers and clinical psychologists. It was also reflected in the work of some sociologists, who were becoming independent methodological leaders in the interdisciplinary project of 'social psychiatry'.
>
> (Pilgrim 2002: 586)

It could be added that the model also provided a theoretical umbrella for the development of multi-disciplinary practice during this period. However, as Pilgrim further points out, the implicit assumption was also that biopsychosocial theory and practice were ultimately under the direction of medically trained doctors. Thus, although it provided space for the articulation of social perspectives, it is questionable whether it ever questioned the hierarchical implications of the older biomedical model. As the more critical challenges of anti-psychiatry and the service user movement emerged (described below), so in some quarters the biopsychosocial model was unable to provide a full accommodation between the more socially oriented radicals and revisionists of the medical model such as Clare. Pilgrim argues that after reaching a high point around 1980 it has become overtaken again by a bioreductionist orthodoxy that has 'returned to medicine', with primary attention given to biology, genetics and drug interventions.

Modernising mental health care – the emergence of new social models

Thus, the reconfiguration of services and the ideological differences that are associated with them are often conflated as being about a dispute between adherence to a 'social' or 'medical' model of mental health. In many ways this is like other reductionist approaches that translate a complex argument into a false duality between two stereotyped alternatives. Today, there are few people who wish to promote in a pure form the Laingian, anti-psychiatric idea that mental disorder does not exist and is a miasma created by the combined forces of capitalism and wicked psychiatrists, or Szasz's (1971) once influential view that mental illness is a form of malingering and therefore a moral issue. On the other hand, if there is a positive legacy of anti-psychiatry, it is the lesson that people who are in mental distress have an authentic voice that should be heard and respected, and that their distress is a form of communication. In addition, it sensitises practitioners to the power relationships through which are defined and applied the categories by which some people are defined as 'normal', and others as sick.

 Rather than think in terms of a single social model, we can identify a range of perspectives or analytical frameworks that can inform the social worker about contexts within which mental distress is experienced, and which provide some indications about appropriate targets of intervention. Chapter 2 provides extended consideration of the main dimensions of the social exclusion of people with mental health problems, but here we consider a range of additional social perspectives that are available to inform the approach of social workers to working in mental health contexts.

Social capital and mental health

Currently, a focus for research and theorising about the relationship between social factors and the incidence of mental distress is the concept of social capital. One of the social scientists associated with the concept is Coleman (1988), who researched linkages between educational outcomes and the social resources available to children, particularly the trustworthiness of the relationships they had with close kinship and neighbourhood networks. Putnam, an American political scientist, drew on Coleman's work in his analysis of local government and civil society in Italy. His work achieved wide influence through his subsequent book on the decline of community solidarity in the US, *Bowling Alone* (2000), which pointed to the apparent decline of social solidarity experienced by people in their communities, the level of engagement they had with voluntary organisations and other societies and the negative consequences of this. The third social theorist associated with the idea of social capital is Bourdieu (1986) who, like Coleman, took his inspiration from the sociology of education, pointing to the benefits that individuals enjoyed where they actively participated in activities that gave them durable networks of social relationships. The common ground, despite methodological and philosophical differences, between Coleman, Putnam and Bourdieu is the idea that membership of and participation in groups or networks builds for individuals resources or 'capital' that can be drawn on to empower people and help them promote their self-interest.

Despite criticisms of the conceptual confusions within the idea of social capital (not least that it is little more than a metaphor which confuses collective resources – the 'social'– with the idea of 'capital' that is inherently individualistic), it has become widely utilised as an approach to thinking about how public health, including mental health, might be improved through engagement by individuals in building trusting relationships within social networks. Examples of where possession of social capital improves mental health outcomes include recovery from drug and alcohol dependence (Webber 2005) or that the existence of social support networks protect against depression (Brown et al., 1986). Finding definitive proof that there is a relationship between those behaviours that build social capital and improvement in mental health has proven beguiling to researchers but difficult to substantiate. Webber (2005) has elegantly identified the difficulties. Most of the research into social capital draws on survey data and this has a number of limitations: simply aggregating details about individuals does not necessarily give an accurate picture of what is happening at community level, a snap shot survey cannot show the direction of causality between whether an absence of social capital causes mental distress, or whether mental distress depletes social capital. There is also a lack of consensus about how social capital can be directly measured, resulting in surveys using proxy indicators, such as voting behaviour or perceptions of community cohesion, with no real clarity as to whether different studies are describing and measuring the same phenomenon.

Box 1.1   Rediscovering community development perspectives in mental health: the *Community Renewal and Mental Health Report*

One of the positive contributions of social capital theory, along with other area-based per-spectives in mental health has been a rediscovery of community development work. A UK report produced by the Kings Fund and the National Institute for Mental Health in England, *Community Renewal and Mental Health*, seeks to identify the working partnerships that can be developed to produce locality-based initiatives to alleviate mental distress and promote well-being (Cameron et al., 2003). This recognises that many of the earlier projects that used community work methods to build alliances with service users and local community groups had become marginalised in the 1990s by a narrower service focus on people experiencing severe mental health problems, while addressing a mental health policy agenda that was increasingly charac-terised by fears of the challenges that mentally ill people were perceived as making to public safety. This was accompanied by measures that brought people with mental health problems into closer association with areas of high deprivation such as moving people with mental health problems into social housing projects where social problems were already concentrated. Stresses arising from living in areas with poor opportunities for leisure, education and employment exacerbated individual problems; and the greater likelihood of experiencing poor physical health in deprived areas also reinforces mental health difficulties. The authors of *Community Renewal and Mental Health* identify a range of opportunities arising from schemes such as urban regeneration partnerships that can enhance economic development and community cohesion in ways that are inclusive of people with, or vulnerable to, mental health problems.

Interest in social capital as a perspective in mental health has now broadened into the concept of 'mental capital'. The UK Government Office for Science's *Foresight Report on Mental Capital and Wellbeing* (Jenkins et al., 2008) systematically reviews the evidence for factors that promote mental health and resilience over the life course:

> Mental capital encompasses both cognitive and emotional resources. It includes people's cog-nitive ability; their flexibility and efficiency at learning; and their 'emotional intelligence', or social skills and resilience in the face of stress. The term therefore captures a key dimension of the elements that establish how well an individual is able to contribute to society and to experience a high quality of life.

> (Beddington et al., 2008: 1057)

'Mental capital' is an attempt to present a holistic perspective that draws together a wide range of cognitive and emotional capacities that individuals may be able to cultivate to maintain their mental health throughout their life. Sceptics may consider that it is another catch-all or rhetorical concept with little analytical precision, but it may nevertheless be a useful umbrella for bringing together approaches that cumulatively could have beneficial effects for the mental well-being of individuals.

Disability theory and the service user movement

Much of the political and theoretical impetus for a new social model has emerged from the disability movement and the development of disability theory (Beresford 2002). It is a significant feature of these developments that, perhaps more than any other area of social theory, this has emerged through 'praxis', the close interaction of political activism and theoretical reflection upon that experience. Key individuals in the development of disability theory such as Mike Oliver, Colin Barnes and Vic Finkelstein are notable for their own personal commitment to activism as well as to building theory. The departure point is generally given as the manifesto of the Union of the Physically Impaired Against Segregation (UPIAS) first adopted in 1974 (Oliver and Barnes 1998). This promoted the argument that disability is not a characteristic of the individual, but is a quality of the physical environment that excludes individuals from social and economic participation. At one level this is a simple observation, and yet such is its potency that it has had profound effects on the academic and political discourses surrounding disability, and provided a significant driver in the development of anti-discriminatory legislation. It has also been a catalyst in the development of a self-aware service user movement that demands to be consulted and to be a stakeholder in the development of services. This also extends to the emergence of user-led research in disability and other fields.

Disability theory, which of course has now gone some way beyond the primary definition of disability as environmental exclusion, although identified with movements of physically disabled people, can also be applied to mental health. Barnes and Bowl (2001) have analysed the service user and survivor-led activism as a 'new social movement' with distinct political strategies:

> The aim is not a redistribution of wealth but to gain control over the discourse within which lives are constructed. These transformative rather than redistributive goals affect the nature of the social action within which contemporary movements are engaged. Contemporary social movements adopt a variety of forms of action which are not based in traditional forms of political participation – such as party membership or political participation – but which utilise a range of sub- and counter-cultural strategies such as festivals, the celebration of alternative life styles, consciousness raising and direct action.
>
> (Barnes and Bowl 2002: 136)

The mental health user-led social movements have been identifiable in the United States and Netherlands since the 1970s. Dutch innovations such as the 'clientenbond', a patient's union established in 1971, and the National Council of Patient Advocates established in 1981, have been significant models for groups in other European countries. A study in England by Wallcraft and Bryant (2003) found many mental health activists consciously saw themselves as part of a broad social movement to empower people who used or had survived the mental health system.

Despite these gains by users and survivors, it is notable that from within 'mainstream' disability theory mental health is not very visible. A 'state of the art' textbook on disability theory contains only two passing references to mental health (Barnes et al., 2002). It seems unfortunate that disability theory offers conceptual ammunition for people working in the mental health field but has not been fully taken on board within the wider disability field as a framework for theory or practice. In an editorial for the *Journal of Mental Health*, Peter Beresford argued for the potential centrality of disability theory as a pillar of a social model of mental health:

> Survivor activists are increasingly considering how such a social model might apply to their situation. There is an interest in developing discussion about the social model of disability to see how it might provide a helpful framework and might need to be adapted for a new 'social model of madness and distress'.

> (Beresford 2002: 583)

As Beresford goes on to argue, the framework of disability theory when applied to mental health shifts terminology from 'crisis intervention', 'acute episodes' and 'breakdown' towards 'support', 'personal assistance' and 'non-medicalised provision'. The visible attainment of this kind of model in the disability field has been the creation of direct payment schemes, now underpinned in the UK by legislation: this gives money directly to those assessed as having needs who can then directly commission their own package of services. However, the barriers to be overcome in moving to this model of provision is indicated by research that finds that within direct payment schemes people with mental health needs are severely under-represented (Ridley and Jones 2003). The implication of the research is that professionals, including social workers, may need to reflect on prevailing assumptions that people in mental distress are inherently unable to make competent choices about their own care.

The recovery model

Also very influential in a number of countries has been a further model which in many respects has been user-led, the recovery movement. Onyett (2003) has commented that, in the face of considerable fragmentation between professionals and user-led perspectives, there has been a surprising convergence around 'recovery' as a unifying perspective. Like so many concepts that are broadly used in mental health, recovery is a contested concept. Ralph and Corrigan (2005) have undertaken some useful teasing out of the concept of recovery and suggest that it has three main usages. The first is the overcoming of symptoms that meet diagnostic criteria for a condition, without any outside intervention. As we will review in relation to severe mental disorders such as schizophrenia, a surprising number of people do manage to make a recovery, against the frequently pessimistic expectations of professionals and lay people alike. The second usage of 'recovery' is to describe the process of improvement and remission of symptoms that results from the purposeful application of treatments that are efficacious. The third usage, and the one that is more prominent in relation to the recovery model as a distinct perspective, is the recovery of hope and purpose on the part of people living with a mental health condition.

The recovery model emerges from a range of historical, theoretical and practice-based perspectives. Sometimes the origin of the recovery perspective is located in the moral treatment movement of the early nineteenth century in Britain as exemplified by the regime developed by John Tuke at the Retreat in York (Roberts and Wolfson 2006). The inspirational affects of first-person narrative accounts of living with mental distress have also been a formative influence (Care Service Improvement Partnership et al., 2007: 3). Allott and Loganathan (2002) cite as a primacy influence the role of Mary Ellen Copeland as a figurehead in the United States, as well as influential practice developments in New Zealand. The recovery literature from the United States tends to focus on the empowerment of the individual; work in New Zealand has often been located within Maori communities and provides a corrective to Western individualism by stressing the importance for recovery of cultural and spiritual factors.

Although there is a longstanding recognition in the clinical literature that many people diagnosed with mental distress experience 'spontaneous remission', this is usually portrayed as being an exception to the generally pessimistic prognosis that characterises medical attitudes. Recovery, as a social perspective in mental health, begins from a basic value position that individuals should be empowered to optimise their own well-being and self-direction:

> Instead of focussing on symptomatology and relief from symptoms, a recovery approach aims to support an individual in their own personal development, building self-esteem, identity and finding a meaningful role in society. Recovery does not necessarily mean restoration of full functioning without support, including medication; it does mean developing appropriate supports and coping mechanisms to be able to deal with mental health experiences rather than being given supports by mental health services, traditionally known as rehabilitation.
>
> (Allott and Loganathan 2002)

Although the recovery model places a strong emphasis on self-determination on the part of people who use services, various commentators have also acknowledged the synergy with some social work approaches such as the strengths perspective (Onyett 2003; Rapp and Wintersteen 1989), for instance, that interventions are based on the principle of user self-determination; the recognition that people with severe and enduring mental health problems retain a capacity for change and self-development; that professional involvement should concentrate on strengths rather than pathology; and that the quality of the relationship between service user and care coordinator is fundamental.

Others have noted the general level of consistency between the recovery model and principles of social work:

> Social work has long-standing experience of person-centred approaches and participative working. Its working principles of empowerment and a rights base are reflected in the specific duties of the approved social worker (Mental Health Act 1983) and most recently expressed in the General Social Care Council *Codes of Practice*.
>
> (Care Service Improvement Parnership et al., 2007: 3)

Box 1.2   Competencies for mental health workers working within a recovery framework

A competent mental health worker:

- understands recovery principles;

- recognises and supports the personal resourcefulness of people with mental illness;

- accommodates diverse views of mental illness, treatments, services and recovery;

- understands and actively protects the rights of people who use services;

- understands discrimination and social exclusion, its impact on people who use services and how to reduce it;

- acknowledges the different cultures and how to work in partnership with them;

- has comprehensive knowledge of community services and resources and actively supports people who use services to use them;

- has knowledge of the 'service user' movement and is able to support its participation;

- has knowledge of family perspectives and is able to support their participation.

(from New Zealand Mental Health Commission, 2001,
cited Care Services Improvement Partnership et al., 2007)

The social models – essential characteristics and future challenges

We have seen that although the development of mental health services in particular countries is shaped by the institutional context, culture and history of welfare of those countries, there has been a very broad convergence towards community-based models of care which embrace to varying degrees elements of social models. Inevitably there is a degree of selectivity in instancing particular models, but it has been suggested that social capital, disability and recovery perspectives are all contributory to those developments. They draw on a range of intellectual and practice-based influences, but it might be argued that they share at least some principles that are core to contemporary social models. A valuable statement of those principles has been set out by Duggan et al. (2002) and the following list draws on their discussion of 'new' social models:

- Many of the problems experienced by people in mental distress are produced by the exclusionary tendencies of social institutions rather than the inherent limitations of those individuals.

- The operation of power is critical in understanding the dynamics of mental health, and social inequality is damaging for health and well-being.

- Social inclusion for people in mental distress is multidimensional and includes their position as producers, consumers, participants and social actors.

- That support should be given to people to recover (and exceed) levels of social functioning and inclusion that they have lost.

- Respect should be given to the voices of people who experience mental distress and the variety of their experiences and identities.

- A needs-based and holistic approach to service delivery requires the development of integrated and joined up services, including those led by service users themselves.

- The quality of life desired by people in mental distress is multifaceted and goes beyond the effects of compliance with pharmacological interventions.

- The evaluation of service quality should incorporate more than professionally defined measures of effectiveness and include outcomes that have been identified by users of services as important.

- The knowledge base for effective service delivery and professional intervention should be pluralistic, incorporating findings from user-led research as well as practice-based evidence.

- The value base for the social model recognises the realisation of autonomy for service users as a basic human need, a concept that goes beyond consumerist conceptions of 'choice'.

For the social models of mental health and their influence upon policy in national contexts – to paraphrase Charles Dickens – it may be the best of times, it may be the worst of times. As was argued earlier in the chapter, there is a resurgence of interest in the social dimensions of mental well-being that is probably stronger than at any time since the highpoints of anti- and critical psychiatry. These models emerge from the 'praxis', the interaction of theory and practice, of alliances of service users, practitioners and academics. It is above all the inclusion of the experience of people living with mental distress that differentiates these models from those earlier movements and intellectual trends.

How these models are being expressed and acted upon is shaped, as we have seen, by the national and institutional contexts in which they develop. This is happening at a historical epoch when welfare states in many countries are experiencing retrenchments and restructuring in response to global and regional economic pressures (Pugh and Gould 2000). These not only constrain the development of services, but they can also add to the very social conditions such as forced migration, unemployment and widening inequality that contribute to mental health problems. Social workers find themselves on the front line supporting individuals and carers who are struggling to overcome mental distress that

Chapter 2

is shaped and reinforced by wider social circumstances. In Chapter 2 we consider in more detail the dynamics of some of these social factors and their implications for mental health social work practitioners.

Activity 1.2 Models of mental health

Refer back to the vignettes at the beginning of this chapter of 'Brian', 'Poppy' and 'Jeremy'. Consider each in terms of the medical, biopsychosocial and social models (including social capital, disability and recovery perspectives) and try to identify which aspects of the three scenarios would be highlighted by the model or perspective. Are there any areas of common ground between the models in their frameworks of understanding of the vignettes?

Key points

- Mental health problems are endemic in most if not all societies and exact a high toll on individuals, families and communities.

- In the latter part of the twentieth century mental health services have moved from large-scale institutions to the community. This has been influenced by a range of factors including cost-saving, developments in pharmacological treatment, public response to hospital-based abuse, and ideological shifts towards a mixed economy of care.

- Social work that operates within a social model does not rule out the possibility that some people have innate vulnerabilities arising from physiological factors, but is informed by evidence that social factors also play a causal role.

- The biopsychosocial model of mental health has been an important intellectual perspective influencing the development of multidisciplinary working in mental health.

- Additional perspectives that inform new social models include social capital, disability theory and the recovery model.

- An overarching perspective from the social perspectives is that many of the problems experienced by people in mental distress are caused by social exclusion from support rather than the inherent limitations of individuals.

Key reading

Care Services Improvement Partnership, Royal College of Psychiatrists and Social Care Institute for Excellence (2007) *A Common Purpose: Recovery in future mental health services, Joint position paper 08*, London: Social Care Institute for Excellence.

Duggan, M. with Cooper, A. and Foster, J. (2002) *Modernising the Social Model in Mental Health: a discussion paper*, London: Social Perspectives Network. Online at http://www.spn.org.uk/fileadmin/SPN_uploads/Documents/Papers/SPN_Papers/spn_paper_1_RP.pdf. Accessed 4 May 2009.

Pilgrim, D. (2002) 'The biopsychosocial model in Anglo-American psychiatry: Past, present and future?', *Journal of Mental Health*, 11(6), 585–594.

2 Developing socially inclusive practice

By the end of this chapter you should have an understanding of:

- Debates around the conceptualisation of social inclusion and exclusion and their relevance to the field of mental health

- The relationship between employment and mental distress, both as a cause and outcome, and evidence-based approaches to supporting people into work

- The causes and prevalence of poverty amongst people with mental health problems

- Reasons for poor physical health amongst many people who have mental health problems

- The significance of accommodation problems for people who have mental health problems and the implications for social work

- Debates around institutional racism and psychiatry and the difficulties for people from black and minority ethnic groups in accessing appropriate services

- The significance of gender as an issue for mental health

- Mental health issues for lesbian, gay and bisexual people

- Key elements of socially inclusive mental health practice.

Dimensions of social exclusion

Systematic reviews of large-scale epidemiological studies in the West find a consistent relationship between rates of mental illness and indicators of social disadvantage, including low income, education, unemployment and low social status (Fryers et al., 2003). Only 24 per cent of people with long-term mental health problems in England are in employment – a smaller proportion than for any other main group of disabled people (Office for National Statistics 2003), and in 2004 over 900,000 people claiming sickness and disability benefit reported mental illness as their primary condition (Office of the Deputy Prime Minister 2004). People with severe mental health problems are three times more likely to be divorced than those without (Meltzer et al., 2002). People with mental health problems are three times more likely to be in debt (Meltzer et al., 2002). Mental illness can create impaired functioning at home, in education or employment, and the restricted life opportunities this produces continue to contribute to poor mental health in an ongoing, self-reinforcing cycle. As a result of the cumulative effect of these associations between mental health problems and social disadvantage, mental health experts have looked increasingly to the concept of social inclusion as an analytical framework to conceptualise this dynamic relationship between social factors and mental distress (Williams 2003; Cameron et al., 2003; Sayce and Curran 2007).

Originating in continental Europe, social exclusion theory asserted that traditional debates around poverty, exemplified by the British tradition of empirical poverty research, overlooked the multidimensional character of the lives of people who were unable to participate in mainstream social activity by virtue of their various deprivations. Social policy analysts tend to identify the origins of the terminology of social exclusion with Lenoir (1974) who used the term 'les exclus' to refer to individuals who fell through social protection systems such as national insurance and whose lives became disconnected from mainstream society. In the 1980s, under French influence, policy-makers at the European Commission began to use the term 'social exclusion' as shorthand for describing multidimensional deprivation, and the term seemed to gather purchase with British Conservative politicians as a sanitised alternative to the discourse of poverty.

Hills et al. (2002) in attempting to offer more analytical precision and a general model of social exclusion, conceptualise the individual as surrounded by a series of contexts, from family and locality going outwards in a series of 'onion rings' to the global economy. The key activities in which a citizen should, if they choose, be able to participate are: consumption (the capacity to purchase goods and services); production (participation in economically or socially valuable activities); political engagement (involvement in local or national decision-making); and social interaction (integration with family, friends and community) (Burchardt et al., 2002: 31). Social exclusion can be summed up in the words of Burchardt (2000) as 'enforced lack of participation' in key social, cultural and political activities.

Compared to social policy as an academic discipline, the mental health literature tends not to be systematic in addressing how mental distress is implicated in these dimensions of social exclusion, but draws on research to show the various pathways through which people experiencing mental distress are often, through process of stigmatisation and powerlessness, disadvantaged in terms of consumption, employment, political engagement and social interaction. A key policy document in this debate has been the Office of the Deputy Prime Minister's report *Mental Health and Social Inclusion* (2004), which synthesised a number of specially commissioned systematic reviews of key variables that were deemed to impact on social inclusion. As one illustration of a cycle of social exclusion it suggests the following:

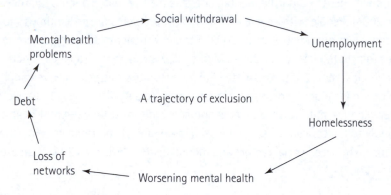

Figure 2.1
Cycle of social exclusion

This is one example of the interaction between social variables and mental disorder. There are many others that could be substituted for this. Morgan et al. (2007) have provided a useful overview of the conceptual and methodological literature on mental health and social exclusion. They point out that research to date attempting to describe and measure the relationship between social exclusion and mental health outcomes or pathways to care tends to draw opportunistically on whatever data are available from surveys or other sources, rather than beginning from models that are well theorised (e.g., Hjern et al., 2004; Webber and Huxley 2004). Despite their shortcomings these studies reveal the multidimensional deprivation of many people with mental health problems and their difficulties in accessing the services that might ameliorate their circumstances. Further studies utilising qualitative approaches are able to draw out the subjective experiences of exclusion lived by people with mental health problems; these studies particularly show the ambiguous and fluctuating nature of exclusion, that people can feel more or less included simultaneously in different areas of their lives – for example, unemployed but supported by friends – and that these experiences change in response to circumstances (Dunn 1999; Parr et al., 2004).

Activity 2.1 Pathways to social exclusion

The *Mental Health and Social Inclusion Report* (Office of the Deputy Prime Minister 2004: 22) recounts 'Liz's story'. Liz worked as a journalist but experienced severe bouts of depression. She was worried about anyone finding out about her mental health problem, and stopped seeing her doctor because she didn't want to take time off work. She explained occasional manic periods as taking time off work. Liz was eventually hospitalised several times. When she tried to go back to work, she couldn't get an interview because of her mental health history. This triggered serious depression and she was detained under the Mental Health Act, and later became homeless.

Consider the diagram in Figure 2.1 showing a typical spiral of mental health problems and social exclusion. What other scenarios can you construct that would illustrate cycles of mental health problems and social exclusion?

Employment

Textbooks on social work and mental health have, in general, not addressed employment and labour market participation as a topic. Yet employment is a social issue that has a profound bearing on the mental health of individuals, as both a cause and a consequence of psychosocial problems, and, as we shall see, more progressive mental health services are increasingly seeing unemployment as part of their remit. Almost half of all people with common mental health problems have taken time off work as a result of their difficulties (Singleton et al., 2001). Prolonged unemployment correlates with deteriorating mental health (Howarth et al., 1998) and, in some cases, suicide (Lewis and Sloggett 1998). Conversely, being in work contributes to symptom reduction, fewer hospital admissions and lower levels of service use (Drake et al., 1999).

Adults with long-term mental health problems have the highest unemployment rate for any of the main groups of disabled people – only 24 per cent of adults with long-term mental health problems are in work (Office for National Statistics 2003; Smith and Twomey 2002). In an unpublished paper for the Department of Work and Pensions, Stickland (cited Tunnard 2004: 19) states that only 10 per cent of those with 'mental illness, phobias and panic attacks' and 23 per cent of those with 'depression and nerve problems' are in employment. Parents with mental health problems will experience labour market disadvantage not only through unemployment but also through 'inadequate employment' (i.e., employment underutilising an individual's capabilities) plus absenteeism and lost earnings for those in work but with a relapsing problem (Rogers and Pilgrim 2003).

Health and social care services spend substantial amounts of money on day and employment services for adults with mental health problems, and there is evidence that many of the individuals who use such services value the support they provide (Office of the Deputy Prime Minister 2004: 54). However, there are also concerns that funding is often locked into outmoded models of employment support that are not socially inclusive, in particular they reinforce dependency rather than movement back into mainstream employment. A number of mental health trusts and social care services still provide or commission sheltered workshops that have high staffing ratios but tend to offer unskilled work with few possibilities for progression and which pay wages at or even below national minimum levels. An alternative model is 'train and place', which provides extended periods of vocational training followed by placement in open employment. There are also 'social firms', sometimes co-operatives, that provide some aspects of sheltered employment but which trade in the open market. Research, including systematic reviews of the evaluation evidence in relation to models of employment support, currently points towards Individual Placement and Support (IPS) as the favoured evidence-based approach (Crowther et al., 2004).

IPS originally developed in the United States, although some British mental health services are now adopting this approach. In some respects the principles on which IPS operates are counter-intuitive and challenge the orthodoxies of traditional sheltered employment. Individuals are supported to find 'real' jobs, not placed in sheltered or intermediate environments. There is minimal emphasis on training, with effort concentrated on the process of job-finding but, once a job has been secured, there is ongoing and time-unlimited support provided to help the person remain in employment. A feature of the model that is important for social workers is that the IPS approach is located within multidis- ciplinary mental health teams so that support for employment can be integrated into the wider processes of care planning, support and therapeutic interventions.

Many voluntary organisations and service user movements have encouraged people with mental health problems to become engaged in voluntary work, advocacy, education and so on. Such activity is regarded as therapeutic and self-empowering. It can also be part of a recovery process leading to paid employment (Aston et al., 2003: 30). However, engagement in unpaid work can result in individuals being called by officers of the Department for Work and Pensions for interviews that involve consideration of prosecution and benefit withdrawal, with negative impacts on their mental health. Governmental determination to deliver employment opportunity for all as a main plank in tackling social exclusion and poverty has led to a number of pilots and programmes to help incapacity benefit recipients to enter, re-enter or remain in paid work. All these are potentially helpful to people with mental health problems and some of the evaluative research that is beginning to emerge points to some of the issues that are relevant to those parents. The most important programmes have been the New Deal for Disabled People (NDDP), the Job Retention and Rehabilitation pilot (JRRP) and Pathways to Work (see Box 2.1).

> **Box 2.1 Lessons from the research evaluations of the New Deal for Disabled People, Job Retention and Rehabilitation Pilot and Pathways to Work**
>
> - People with mental health problems need access to more specialist help and support than is provide by generic unemployment services (Corden et al., 2005).
>
> - The attitudes of employers towards people with mental health problems need to be modified. Many employers hold the view that mental illness is a particularly difficult area of disability (Aston et al., 2003).
>
> - GPs also need to be more understanding of mental health and employment; they have limited awareness of services to support return to work, and that sickness certification and work rehabilitation are under-resourced aspects of GPs' work (Mowlam and Lewis 2005).
>
> - The increased emphasis within the benefit system on so-called work-focused interviews has unintended consequences for many people with mental health problems (Corden et al., 2005); they may have a range of apprehensions, including aversion to dealing with mail, fear of travelling, social phobias, which may lead them to fail to attend interviews with consequential possible reduction in their benefit. Though the interview regulations state that sanctions should not be applied to illness-related behaviour, there is considerable scope for discretion by officers and no right of review.

Poverty

There is extensive research showing the correlation between the experience of poverty and mental health problems (see for example Whitley et al., 1999; Weich et al., 2001; Payne 2006). While we should avoid over-generalising the individual experiences of users of mental health services, and thereby adding to their stigmatisation, it is generally recognised that various forms of mental disorder impact on the economic welfare of individuals. Financial hardship and insecurity are sources of stress, which in turn is a contributory factor to the onset and severity of mental illness. There are several reasons why experiencing a mental disorder compromises people's capabilities in maintaining their income and financial independence. They may be unable to retain a job, or face stigmatisation in securing employment (see above). Individuals may have temporary or enduring impairments in their cognitive capacity to deal with financial affairs (for example, depression can impair someone's concentration and problem-solving capabilities). Also, many mental disorders are fluctuating in their severity, or have patterns of remission and relapse, which adds to the complexity of individuals' needs and capabilities to manage.

Over and above factors that arise directly from mental distress, there is also substantial evidence that there are structural factors – for instance, located in social security systems, financial services and work practices – that also contribute to poverty among people with mental health problems (see Davis 2003; Plumpton and Bostock 2003; Citizens' Advice Bureau 2004). There are longstanding and unresolved debates as to the relative merits of 'social selection theories' that suggest that people who are prone to mental disorders drift downward into poverty, thereby further increasing their risk for mental illness, contrasted with 'social causation theories' implying a direct causal relationship between poverty and the triggering of mental illness. Whatever the relative merits of these positions (see Costello et al., 2003; Rutter 2003), some general statements can be made about the vulnerability of people with mental health problems to financial adversity and poverty. These have been usefully summarised by Davis (2003):

- Poverty impacts directly on the individual's mental health and well-being.

- A high proportion of people with mental health problems are unemployed and are dependent on state benefits.

- A history or current status of mental ill-health can lead to obstacles in accessing financial services, with higher levels of refusal of credit.

- Using mental health services (such as long-term or 'revolving door' hospital admissions) increases the complexities encountered by individuals in managing their incomes.

- The cognitive impairments produced by mental illness increase the challenges and complexity of securing entitlements to benefits and managing personal finances.

It is also becoming evident from research that the effect of poverty on mental health is not just an effect of absolute poverty, it is also a function of inequality and relative poverty, that is, people on lower incomes are more likely to experience common mental disorders if they live in areas of greater income inequality (Weich et al., 2001). It seems that the stress of poverty is amplified by the awareness of the relative affluence of others (Wilkinson 2001).

A primary reason for poverty amongst people with mental health problems is that they are dependent for their income on social security benefits. Over 900,000 adults in England claim sickness and disability benefits for mental health conditions; this group is larger than the total number of unemployed people claiming Jobseekers' Allowance in England (Office of the Deputy Prime Minister 2004). Parents relying on long-term benefits because they are unable to work because of a mental health problem will be claiming an incapacity benefit. The main incapacity benefits involved are Incapacity Benefit, Severe Disablement Allowance and Income Support with a disability premium. Based on unpublished data supplied to the author by the Department of Work and Pensions, at May 2005 there were 198,900 parents in receipt of these benefits who had a 'mental and behavioural disorder' as defined by the World Health Organization's *ICD-10* (Gould 2006c). These parents were in turn responsible for the care of at least 368,000 children, showing that mental health is implicated in the wider issue of family poverty, and that political objectives of eliminating child poverty have to address the problems of adult mental health (Gould 2006c).

Analysis of the Labour Force Survey longitudinal datasets shows that the onset of mental health problems significantly increases the risk of employment loss, compared to other health conditions or impairments (Burchardt 2003). The number of people coming into Incapacity Benefit citing mental health problems as their main disability almost doubled between 1995 and 2004, from 475,000 to 848,000 (Office of the Deputy Prime Minister 2004: 62). Consequently, mechanisms and rules relating to returning to work and entitlement to benefits are critically important for families where a member has a mental health problem. The government's increasing emphasis on 'conditionality' of entitlement to welfare benefits, that is, creating additional tests of whether an individual is unfit or unable to work, adds to the strain on their mental health.

Physical health

Concentration on the social inequalities directly associated with mental health problems can draw attention from the very significant disadvantages in relation to physical health which are experienced by people with mental health problems. The mental health charity Rethink has collated statistics relating to people living with schizophrenia and bipolar disorder suggesting that they experience, compared to people without mental health problems: two to four times the rate of cardiovascular disease, two to four times the rate of respiratory disease, five times the rate of diabetes, eight times the rate of hepatitis C, and fifteen times the rate of HIV (Rethink 2008). Not surprisingly in the light of these figures, there is for people with severe mental health problems a higher risk of premature death, estimated in the government White Paper *Choosing Health* as 1.5 times a greater likelihood, and this is after controlling for suicide (Department of Health 2004a):

> People with severe mental illness (SMI) are 1.5 times more likely to die prematurely than those without; partly due to suicide, but also to death from respiratory and other diseases. Depression is consistently been linked to mortality following a myocardial infarction; it increases the risk of heart disease fourfold, even when other risk factors like smoking are controlled for. People with severe mental illnesses also tend to have a poor diet; they are more likely to be obese; to smoke more; to access routine health checks less frequently, and get less health promotion input than the general population.

> (Department of Health 2004a: 132)

On average people diagnosed with schizophrenia live for ten years less than the general population, some of this will be attributable to high-risk behaviour and suicide, but this disparity is mainly attributable to physical health problems (Allebeck 1989).

Some of the physical health difficulties associated with mental health problems are related to lifestyle behaviours that occur when individuals have reduced levels of motivation, perhaps caused by depression or negative symptoms of schizophrenia. People with severe mental health problems tend to eat less well, smoke more heavily and take less exercise than the general population (Phelan et al., 2001), and these factors contribute to higher levels of cardiovascular disease (McCreadie and Kelly 2002). They are three times more likely than the general population to have an alcohol dependency problem (Institute of Alcohol Studies 2003). Smoking is a particular issue for people with mental health problems, and this has been recognised in the delayed implementation in mental health inpatient units of anti-smoking legislation: adults with common mental health problems are twice as likely to smoke (Coultard et al., 2000) and deaths from smoking-related disease are twice as high amongst people with schizophrenia (McNeill 2001).

Sometimes the level of causality is in the other direction, with physical health problems leading to mental health difficulties; for instance, receiving a diagnosis of cancer or heart disease may contribute to problems of depression and anxiety (Royal College of Psychiatry 2009). Research suggests that approximately 70 per cent of new cases of depression in older people are attributable to physical health problems (Evans et al., 2003). Box 2.2 presents a summary of the reasons why the health risks are so high for people with mental health problems.

Box 2.2   Why are the health risks for people with mental health problems so high?

The following summary is from a report by Rethink (2008):

- *Problems of gaining access to physical health care.* Many inpatient facilities for people with mental health problems do not have links to general practice, so physical health problems are less likely to be attended. Where people with mental health problems are located in the community, GP practices can sometimes be perceived as unresponsive and unwelcoming.

- *'Diagnostic overshadowing.'* This expression is sometimes used to describe the situation where people known to have mental health problems present to their GP with a physical symptom, but this is interpreted as a manifestation of their mental disorder such as depression or anxiety. The physical condition may go undiagnosed, or not be picked up until it has worsened, and treatment may then be more urgent or complicated.

- *Gaps between services.* Mental health specialists may lack expertise in areas of physical illness, and sometimes the converse may be the case, resulting in neither service taking responsibility for the holistic care of the individual. Sometimes people with mental health problems may also find themselves caught up in 'boundary disputes', where services argue about who has primary responsibility for an individual.

- *Lifestyle and poverty.* Low income is associated with smoking and with nutritionally deficient diets, both of which are associated with some of the health complications discussed above. People with mental health problems may also be less likely to respond to health promotion campaigns that would improve lifestyle and diet.

- *Medication problems.* Many drugs that are prescribed for mental health problems have physical side effects such as weight gain, or may raise the risks of developing conditions such as diabetes.

- *Disempowerment and lack of confidence.* The cumulative effect of interaction with services that individuals perceive as insensitive or rejecting may be to inculcate feelings of dis-empowerment and pessimism in people with mental health problems. This can lead to a downward spiral where individuals are reluctant to take the initiative in demanding their entitlement to proper treatment for physical conditions.

Housing

For human beings one of the main anchors of their feelings of well-being and security is to have adequate shelter or housing. Not only is this a precondition for physical health, it also contributes to psychological security and is the base from which individuals and families are able to participate in community life, whether it be children attending school regularly, or adults holding down employment. Yet once again, this basic need is one of the dimensions on which people with mental health problems fare poorly compared to the rest of the population. This is reflected in the physical condition of their accommodation, the lack of security they experience in tenure of their homes and their over-representation amongst the homeless population. As with other aspects of social exclusion such as unemployment and poverty, the causal relationship between housing difficulties and mental health problems operate in either direction: housing accommodation problems contribute to mental health problems, and people with mental health problems are more likely to experience difficulties with their accommodation.

The Office for National Statistics census of psychiatric morbidity (Meltzer et al., 2002) found that, compared to the general population, people with mental health problems were:

- one and a half times more likely to live in rented housing with higher uncertainty about their security of tenure;

- twice as likely to express dissatisfaction with their accommodation or that the state of repair is poor;

- four times more likely to say that their health had been made worse by their housing situation.

The social and psychological mechanisms that connect housing to mental health were explored in Brown and Harris's (1978) classic study of depression amongst working-class women where housing – its location, repair, size and neighbours – was a vulnerability factor. Since deinstitutionalisation and care in the community, people with mental health problems have found themselves living in a multiplicity of housing situations, although it should not be overlooked that most people with mental health problems do live in mainstream provision, that is, less than 20 per cent live in specialist accommodation provided by voluntary organisations, health and social care providers, local authorities or housing associations (Weich and Lewis 1998, cited Office of the Deputy Prime Minister 2004). Of the 80 per cent who live in mainstream accommodation, that is, owning or renting their own home, 50 per cent live alone; of course for some of these individuals this is a preference, but the statistic is probably also a proxy for the isolation that accompanies many who have mental health problems.

Social workers who work with people with mental health problems need to be able to help people navigate their way through the legal and funding frameworks which determine their housing entitlements, or at least to be able to signpost people towards expert help. Rebecca Pritchard (2006) has commented on the deficits in social work training in relation to this area of policy and practice, despite the demonstrated level of housing need amongst mental health service users. Practitioners would be better able to support individuals if they have a working knowledge of the 2002 Homelessness Act, which defines the social groups that can be considered to have 'priority need' for being accommodated by the local authority. Research indicates that about 9 per cent of those accepted for priority need have a mental health problem (Office of the Deputy Prime Minister 2004). However, the recognition of the problem does not necessarily lead to a solution: often this results in placement in temporary, unsuitable accommodation. Alternatively, people who are living in hostels or inpatient units can find themselves in a 'Catch 22' situation, accommodated in such placements beyond the point where this is appropriate to their mental health needs, because they are not viewed as sufficiently high priority (Tarpey and Watson 1997, cited office of the Deputy Prime Minister 2004). Again, Rebecca Pritchard (2006) points to the need for social workers to develop skills in joint working with other agencies to facilitate appropriate placements and to seek to influence the local Homelessness Strategy which is statutorily required of local authorities.

Many individuals with severe mental health needs slip through the net of services and become homeless. A simplistic characterisation of homeless people with mental health problems is that they are casualties of the closure of long-term hospital beds, ex-patients who find themselves on the streets, but with the passing of time since the closure of asylums it is clear that many homeless individuals never were long-stay patients and have followed other pathways to homelessness. The research has been usefully reviewed by Redmond (2005). A study of homeless men in four UK cities found that 41 per cent of them had an identified mental illness prior to losing their homes (Crane 1999). Often a significant life event such as the death of a close relative or breakdown of a relationship had exacerbated mental health problems and capacity for coping, leading to leaving or loss of the home. Some studies suggest that schizophrenia is particularly implicated in this dynamic of crisis and homelessness (Redmond 2005).

The experience of homelessness itself can also (unsurprisingly) precipitate mental health problems. Loss of a home is almost inevitably likely to trigger feelings of despair, low self-esteem and, ultimately, depression. One US study found that one-third of homeless people had mental health problems that had not existed prior to losing their homes; within this group almost one-third had been in care as children, an indicator of the precarious social status of this group of young people (Sullivan et al., 2000). Alcohol and drug misuse can also be a complicating factor for homeless people with mental health problems, and has been estimated to be three to five times higher than for the non-homeless population (Williams and Avebury 1995). For some people their problems with alcohol and drugs may pre-date and be a precipitating factor in their homelessness, for others it is a response to the distress

Chapter 6

of their homeless situation. In both instances it is a complicating factor for both their physical and their mental health. Dual diagnosis involving schizophrenia and substance misuse (further discussed in Chapter 6) is particularly prevalent in studies of homeless populations (10–20 per cent in the US according to Breaky (1996)).

There are innumerable examples of models of supported accommodation, re-housing initiatives and outreach projects to help people with housing and mental health problems , and many such enterprises will be able to cite instances of individuals who have been helped back into stable and secure living situations. However, this field is bedevilled by an absence of rigorous evaluation studies to identify which are the most effective kinds of intervention for which service user group (Chilvers et al., 2006; Webber 2008).

Mental health, identity and inequality

'Race', ethnicity and mental health

It is now widely accepted that members of black and minority ethnic groups receive discriminatory treatment in relation to mental health services, to the extent that psychiatry is described by some as 'institutionally racist' (Sashidharan 2001). Critics such as Suman Fernando (1991) have pointed to the ways in which the history of psychiatry as a medical discipline reflects the cultural assumptions of dominant post-imperialist cultures. Thus, psychiatry has historically characterised peoples from the African and Indian continents in particular as innately less emotionally and psychologically sophis- ticated than Western people, and more driven by biological, physical urges. The effects, it is argued, of psychiatry as an institutionally racist discipline has been that people from black and minority ethnic groups are over-represented in services which are coercive, particularly compulsory admissions to mental hospitals, and under-represented as users of mental health services that are designed to be supportive or preventative.

This perspective is reinforced by statistics in relation to patterns of service use. In 2005 the Department of Health launched a five-year programme to improve services for black and minority ethnic groups (*Delivering Race Equality in Mental Health Care*), which included an annual survey of inpatients called

Count Me In (Commission for Healthcare Audit and Inspection 2007). The following results are derived from the 2007 survey, but these are not significantly at variance from the 2005 and 2006 figures. Admissions were higher than average among several minority ethnic groups for both genders – particularly in the Black Caribbean, Black African, Other Black, White/Black Caribbean Mixed and White/Black African Mixed groups – with rates of over three times higher than average, and over ten times higher in the Other Black group. There were 43 percent of patients admitted compulsorily under a section of the Mental Health Act, and again certain groups were over-represented: rates of detention were higher than the national average among the Black Caribbean, Black African, Other Black and White/Black Caribbean Mixed groups (by 19 per cent to 38 per cent), and detention under section 37/41 (imposed by courts) was also higher in these groups (except Black African). Other research studies show that once members of black and minority ethnic groups do engage with services they are less likely to be offered therapeutic interventions, and more likely to be treated with drugs (Chen et al., 1991) or other physical interventions such as ECT (Shaikh 1985).

The observation that over-representation is a feature in the compulsorily detained population being matched by under-representation at earlier points in the care process is again supported by the *Count Me In* 2007 data. Within the Black Caribbean, Black African and Other Black groups, rates of referral from GPs and community mental health teams were lower than the national average, and rates of referral from the criminal justice system were higher than average in the Black Caribbean and Other Black groups. The Other White group also had lower rates of referral from GPs and community mental health teams. This picture tends to corroborate qualitative research which suggests a cycle whereby members of some black and ethnic minority groups only come onto the radar of mental health services at points of crisis and after opportunities for preventative engagement have been missed. This is compounded by the apprehension of some members of black and minority ethnic groups that engagement with mental health services will elicit a coercive response. This dynamic of avoidance and compulsion has been described in the research study *Breaking the Circles of Fear* (Sainsbury Centre for Mental Health 2002).

Attempts from within psychiatry to explain mental health inequalities between ethnic groups have been through several stages. 'Transcultural psychiatry' saw difference as explained by the failure of Western psychiatry to develop diagnostic categories and methods of assessment that were sufficiently attuned to the diversity of cultural beliefs and norms. Essentially, this was an attempt to use anthropological methods of understanding the exotic nature of foreign cultures and elaborating the concepts used by Western psychiatry so that they could be applied across cultures, rather than critically deconstructing the practice of psychiatry itself. As an example, in the 1980s the work of Philip Rack (1982), a Bradford-based psychiatrist, became influential amongst practitioners which proposed a culturally competent approach that used 'insights' about the culture of minority ethnic groups to assist practitioners in working with members of these groups. Thus, it was argued that depression was under-diagnosed among the members of Pakistani communities because they supposedly expressed their emotional distress in terms of physical symptoms, such as vague abdominal pains, and so on. The implication of this approach is always that non-European cultures have some kind of deficit in relation to their experience and communication of mental distress. A more sophisticated version of this anthropological approach is found in Littlewood and Lipsedges' *Aliens and Alienists* (1997), which locates intercultural misunderstanding of mental health in the ethnic diversity of mental health professionals (e.g., Indian psychiatrists basing treatment decisions about a Polish patient on the assessment made by a Malaysian nurse), and in the alienation and distress of members of disempowered minorities such as young male African Caribbeans. Such approaches represented liberal attempts to acknowledge the differential levels of treatment offered to members of black and minority ethnic groups, but without directly addressing power and racism as dimensions of mental health practice.

Some psychiatrists, understandably, dispute the assertion that mental health services are institutionally racist (for example, Singh and Burns 2006). Their arguments draw on research showing that higher rates of psychosis are consistently found in UK community-based epidemiological surveys, using validated diagnostic instruments (e.g. Bhugra and Bhui 2001), and international research showing that higher rates of psychosis are found across the world amongst migrant populations, regardless of colour and ethnicity (Cantor-Graae and Selten 2005). Singh and Burns cite research indicating that there are cultural differences between families in their manner of seeking intervention when a member is mentally distressed, with African Caribbean families contacting the police, whereas Indian or Pakistani families bring their difficulties to the health services. They also cite research suggesting that African Caribbean people are more likely to be compulsorily admitted the more chronic is their condition: a spiral of disengagement from services over time. Singh and Burns argue that the description of mental health services as institutionally racist demoralises well-meaning practitioners and reinforces the problems of engaging with members of black and minority ethnic groups, so becoming a self-fulfilling prophecy. However, it is arguable that the evidence they cite for their arguments – increasing avoidance of services over time and avoidance of services by families – could equally be instanced as evidence for the 'circles of fear' hypothesis.

The debates about race and mental health practice also need to reflect the increasing urgency of the problems experienced by asylum seekers, refugees and displaced people whose numbers, globally, are rising inexorably. Many of these people become detained while their status is reviewed by immigration authorities, despite frequently having experienced profound trauma and stress. A systematic review of research studies of mental health outcomes for immigration detainees found high levels of mental health problems (Robjant et al., 2009). Anxiety, depression and post-traumatic stress disorder were commonly experienced, as were self-harm and suicidal thinking; many of these outcomes persist beyond release from detention. These outcomes were present in adults, young people and children, with clear implications that social workers who work with asylum seekers and refugees of all ages need to engage with their mental health needs.

Gender

Since the 1960s and the 'first wave' of feminism, women's mental health has been a topic of considerable interest to social researchers and theorists. The particular focus of debate has been the predominance of women not only in the inpatient psychiatric population, but particularly in community-based epidemiological studies which have consistently found higher rates, relative to men, of depression and other so-called common mental disorders. It is generally found that prevalence rates for psychotic conditions – primarily schizophrenia and bipolar disorder – are broadly equal for men and women, so depression in particular has become the main subject of debate in relation to gender inequalities and mental health.

The attempts to explain these inequalities have taken various turns. The 'social causation' argument takes these differences in the experienced levels of depression between and women as real, that is, women do suffer measurably higher levels of mental distress, and seeks to explain this in terms of social pressures that operate differentially on women. An influential contribution to this perspective came from the research of Walter Gove (1972), which pointed to the higher levels of depression amongst married women, compared to single women, whereas married men experienced lower levels of depression than single men. This has been taken to be an indicator that women are relatively disadvantaged within heterosexual partnerships; that marriage acts as a protective factor for men but as a risk for women. Also influential (and cited at various points throughout this book) was the research by Brown and Harris (1978) into the social basis of depression amongst working-class women in the London borough of Camberwell. This study showed the vulnerability to depression that was generated by various social factors, some of which are gendered, such as caring for three or more children under 14, lack of a confiding relationship with a (male) partner, and lack of employment outside the home. Within the Brown and Harris model these vulnerabilities become the precondition for depression which may be triggered by negative life events such as divorce or bereavement. Feminist scholarship continued to add to the social causation thesis, citing the vulnerabilities of women to depression when their self-esteem was impaired or they encountered oppressive life circumstances such as domestic violence.

An alternative explanatory framework for accounting for the prevalence of women in mental health statistics has been the 'social constructionist' perspective. This perspective actually encompasses a range of theories. There is a body of research into help-seeking behaviour which finds that men and women communicate distress in different ways. Dohrenwend and Dohrenwend (1977) found that women are more ready than men to acknowledge unhappiness, to articulate their distress in psychological terms, and to be ready to engage with treatment for their mental condition. The corollary of this is evidence that men deny their distress, or communicate it in physical and behavioural modes such as antisocial behaviour or substance misuse, thereby accounting for their predominance in crime statistics and prevalence rates for alcohol and drug dependency. Men are also over-represented within diagnostic categories which are defined in terms of antisocial behaviour, such as psychopathy. The research into pathways to mental health care also find that medical practitioners are more likely to label women as having mental health problems than men (Goldberg and Huxley 1980). This finding appears to provide supportive evidence for researchers that mental health practitioners typically operationalise judgements as to what constitutes mental health and well-being that are biased towards typically male attributes (Broverman et al., 1970). This potentially generates a 'Catch 22' situation for women whereby if they conform to male stereotypes of female behaviour, they may be labelled as mentally unwell, whereas if they reject the traditional woman's role, this may also be seen as pathological. This constructionist perspective is augmented by the work of cultural historians such as Showalter (1987) who draw attention to the historical preoccupations of the founding fathers (sic) of psychiatry, who seemed obsessed with the control of women's sexuality, and the construction of gender-laden diagnostic categories such as hysteria.

More recent sociological analysis of gender and mental health statistics remind us that gender is highly confounded by association with other key social variables such as social class, educational background and social circumstances (Rogers and Pilgrim 2003). Some of the apparent 'excess' of depressive illness amongst women is less apparent when these variables are controlled for. It is also useful to remind ourselves that the Brown and Harris study, though it has been so influential in the discourse around gender and depression, does not compare women with men; the researchers focused on women for reasons of convenience, that they were more likely to be available during the day to participate in lengthy research interviews (Brown and Harris 1978: 48, cited Rogers and Pilgrim 2003).

Though the main focus of research into gender has been the over-representation of women in mental health statistics, there seems to be an increasing recognition of the issues facing men. The exception to the relative silence in relation to men has been a substantial body of research showing the damaging impact of unemployment on their mental health (see above). The emergence of interest in men's mental health is also in relation to the relatively high suicide rates among young men, some of which are accounted for by severe depression and psychosis (Appleby et al., 1999). There is also a growing evidence-base for higher levels of sexual abuse of boys than had previously been recognised, and the adverse mental health outcomes associated with this, again including higher rates (as many as ten times) the level of suicidality in the general population (see O'Leary and Gould 2008).

Lesbians, gay men and bisexuals and mental health

There are a range of mental health issues that have only relatively recently begun to be acknowledged and researched that relate to people who are lesbian, gay or bisexual (LGB) (King et al., 2008). There is now a growing body of evidence that shows how discrimination against people on the basis of their sexual orientation contributes to higher levels of mental health problems. The difficulties of LGB people have been compounded by the historical pathologisation by psychiatry of homosexuality, both in psychological theories such as psychoanalysis that regarded attraction between members of the same sex as deviant, and in psychiatric diagnostic approaches that similarly categorised homosexuality as a mental disorder. Homosexuality was not declassified from the Diagnostic and Statistical Manual of Mental Disorders until 1973, and from the International Statistical Classification of Diseases and Related Health Problems until 1992 (Fawcett and Karban 2005). Inpatient treatment, sometimes using aversion therapy to 'cure' people of homosexuality, persisted into the 1970s and, in the UK, sexuality as a legal ground for compulsory detention in hospital was not excluded until the 1983 Mental Health Act.

The largest research study to date of rates of mental illness amongst lesbian women, gay men and bisexual people (amongst what the authors refer to as a 'dearth' of research in this area) found higher rates of mental disorder as detected by CIS-R, a validated screening instrument, compared to the general population, and high levels of planned and actual self-harm (Warner et al., 2004). A review of the international literature confirmed that LGB people are at significantly higher risk than heterosexual people of suicidal feelings, self-harm, drug or alcohol misuse and having a mental health problem (King et al., 2008). The findings were generally similar for men and women. However, lesbian and bisexual women were at particular risk of suicidal feelings and drug or alcohol dependence, while gay and bisexual men were over four times more likely than heterosexual men to attempt suicide (King et al., 2008).

Explanations for these higher risks to the mental health problems of LGB people focus on the negative impacts of homophobic discrimination. For example, the Warner et al., study (2004) found that suicidality for women was associated with having been insulted at school and having been assaulted during the previous five years. The majority of this sample (83 per cent) had experienced damage to property, physical attacks or verbal bullying. Attention has been drawn to the negative psychological impact of 'internalised homophobia', where the experience of negative social reactions and discrimination contribute to feelings of low self-esteem and even self-hatred (Stonewall 2008).

Although social attitudes towards sexual orientation has been changing, and legislation has supported the formal rights of LGB people, surveys into their experience of mental health services finds some evidence of the persistence of unsympathetic attitudes. A survey conducted by MIND and researchers from University College London (Warner et al., 2004) found that the main issues for LGB people in relation to mental health services were encountering:

* mixed or negative reactions when being open about their sexuality with health professionals;

* a lack of empathy around sexuality issues on the part of health professionals;

* visible discomfort on the part of health professionals, and deliberate attempts to avoid discussing sexuality;

* the assumption that all service users are heterosexual;

* the assumption that being gay, lesbian or bisexual must be a problem for LGB service users;

* a minority of health professionals still make a causal link between homosexuality and mental ill health;

* a minority of health professionals still display overt homophobia.

Consequently, some LGB people express a preference for seeking support from practitioners who themselves self-identify as gay, lesbian or bisexual, or may choose to refer themselves to an organisation that explicitly serves the LGB population. King and McKeown (2003) have made the case for training for mental health practitioners to change their attitudes and approach to working with people of differing sexual orientation, so that mainstream services are more accessible and helpful.

Building socially inclusive mental health practice

The relevance of developing approaches to practices that encourage and reinforce the social inclusion of people with mental health problems has been steadily moving up the policy agenda. In 2007 the Department of Health published a report, *Capabilities for Inclusive Practice*, which attempts to draw out the generic principles applicable to all mental health professionals and service delivery organisations 'intended to be a resource for reflection, challenge and practice change' (Department of Health 2007a: 3). Its key aspects are summarised in Box 2.3.

Box 2.3 Key aspects of inclusive practice as identified in Capabilities for Inclusive Practice (Department of Health 2007a)

Socially inclusive mental health practitioners should:

- *Work in partnership.* Compared with traditional services, staff resources are invested and more time is dedicated to building relationships with people in community organisations. Identify and challenge discriminatory attitudes and practices towards people with mental health issues. Promote awareness of and uphold service users' rights to access all organisations.

- *Respect diversity.* Undertake specific searches for community resources which are targeted at minority and under-served groups (search for resources that target minority and under-served groups, whether or not they have a mental health difficulty).

- *Practise ethically.* Understand the importance of informal relationships, strengths and aspirations in the service user's recovery process and show this in assessment and planning processes, such as through the Care Programme Approach. Provide information, opportunities to visit and try out participation in a variety of community settings, along with personalised support, so that people with mental health problems can make informed choices about their own community participation within a wider approach to empowerment.

- *Challenge inequality.* Demonstrate an understanding of people with mental health problems, particularly as this relates to access to community inclusion. This includes recognition of the feelings of distress and shame that can be caused by discrimination and how negative

---

reputations can develop and be sustained, and how they can be dismantled. Recognise the processes of ignorance, fear, abuse of power, stigmatisation and institutional discrimination within communities that lead to the exclusion of people with mental health issues.

- *Support recovery.* Support service users to clarify their aspirations, celebrate their successes, find strength in their resilience in the face of adversity, tackle their mental health problems and plan their recovery journeys (as revealed in assessment and care planning documentation).

- *Identify people's needs and strengths.* Documentation and practice in initial assessments, eligibility decisions and reviews of intervention pays attention to people's life ambitions and current assets. This includes a focus on job retention and retention of other roles and relationships, especially in early intervention, crisis resolution and inpatient services.

- *Provide service user centred care.* Work positively and creatively with the service user and their family, including at those times when their goals are in conflict. Assess the individual qualities of each community opportunity. Support service users to participate in mainstream community settings to a maximum extent as a full and equal member of the setting.

- *Make a difference.* Service users themselves often report that practitioners focus on limitations and weaknesses when developing care plans. This approach is a wasted opportunity as there is a richness of information to be gathered from understanding the health and inclusive elements of an individual's current life, their aspirations and previous successes. A repertoire of knowledge and skills will be required to facilitate a socially inclusive approach and to ensure that appropriate resources are accessed and that the service user experiences optimum choice. Practitioners must endeavour to maintain an up-to-date knowledge base of evidence-based interventions, NICE Guidelines and best practice and should evaluate its integration into their practice.

- *Promote safety and positive risk taking.* Acknowledge and respond to the trauma and distress caused by exclusion. Include 'risk of exclusion' in risk assessments by ensuring that risk assessments are hopeful rather than pessimistic, informed by the service user's ambitions and increase rather than decrease opportunities for recovery and a valued lifestyle. In this way, the principle of the 'least restrictive alternative' is complemented with the principle of the 'most inclusive alternative'.

- *Continue personal development and learning.* Develop several possible explanations for what is happening in the service user's life and reflect on these. Understand competing definitions, philosophies and practices of inclusion and recognise the competition between inclusion and other viewpoints and priorities. As needed, work in a wide variety of community locations rather than just in one office or workplace.

It has been argued in the first two chapters of this book that there is a re-emergence of social perspectives in mental health, and that although the facets of this are diverse, overall they suggest an outlook for social work practice that differs in a number of respects from traditional 'clinical' approaches. It acknowledges that the operation of power is critical in understanding the dynamics of mental health. Social work has an established tradition of working in anti-discriminatory and anti-oppressive ways, more developed than in the other mental health professions (Fernando 1991) and this is a contribution that social work brings to the wider development of mental health practice in multi-disciplinary settings. Also, rediscovery of the community and locality as contexts within which mental health and distress are experienced also re-assert community development as a legitimate aspect of social work practice, alongside individual psychosocial interventions.

In summary, if social work is to take inclusion of people in mental distress seriously as a framework for practice, then some broadening of our view of the scope of social work is required. Taking Hill et al.'s (2002) model of social inclusion, service users need to be seen in the round as producers, consumers, participants and social actors, not just as passive recipients of services. In relation to 'production' or employment, it means closer involvement in brokerage of job-finding and retention, an area that has not only been outside the training and education of British social workers, but also traditionally disdained as outside the remit of professional practice as traditionally conceived. As Jordan has commented generally about contemporary social work, it will need to 'take a broader view of its remit, to include economic activity, social regeneration, community work and many projects and units that do not at present think of themselves in its terms' (Jordan and Jordan 2000). If social work does not respond to these challenges, then the possibility is that its role in relation to social inclusion will be colonised by other newly emerging occupational groups, such as the Department of Work and Pension's 'personal advisers' within government employment agencies, who have little training in mental health or psychosocial interventions (Gould 2006a).

Key points

- Although the terms 'social inclusion' and 'social exclusion' are contested within the social sciences, they are useful conceptual tools for analysing the inequalities that affect people with mental health problems.

- There is a strong correlation between experiencing mental health problems and lack of employment or underemployment. This relationship can be causal with unemployment leading to a range of psychological difficulties and, conversely, people with mental health problems find it difficult to re-enter employment.

- People with mental health problems experience disproportionate levels of poverty, arising from a variety of factors including dependency on welfare benefits, lack of secure employment, and the difficulties of accessing financial services.

- People with mental health problems also experience adverse physical health because of higher exposure to lifestyle factors associated with poor health, side effects of pharmacological treatments and difficulties in accessing physical health care.

- Disadvantage is experienced by people with mental health problems in relation to the quality and security of their accommodation.

- Psychiatry continues to be accused of institutional racism, with people from several black and minority ethnic groups being over-represented in relation to coercive interventions and under-represented as beneficiaries of supportive interventions.

- Women are over-represented in several categories of mental disorder, particularly mood disorders, which reflects both social inequality and, it is argued, gender biases within psychiatric taxonomies and mental health practice.

- Latterly it has begun to be recognised that lesbian, gay and bisexual people experience high levels of mental distress, much of it related to the negative impacts of homophobic discrimination.

Key reading

Office of the Deputy Prime Minister (2004) *Mental Health and Social Exclusion: Social Exclusion Unit Report*, London: Office of the Deputy Prime Minister.

Rogers, A. and Pilgrim, D. (2003) *Mental Health and Inequality*, Basingstoke: Palgrave Macmillan.

Sayce, L. and Curran, C. (2007) 'Tackling social exclusion across Europe' in Knapp, M., McDaid, Mossialos, E. and Thornicroft, G. (eds), *Mental Health Policy and Practice Across Europe*, Maidenhead: Open University Press.

3 The social work role in mental health services

By the end of this chapter you should have an understanding of:

- The historical debates around the transition from institution- to community-based care

- The policies and processes that have influenced the integration of mental health services

- The place of social work within multidisciplinary mental health teams

- The role of care management and the Care Programme Approach in mental health

- Implications of the 'personalisation agenda' and direct payments for mental health services

- The role of social work in 'new' mental health services, including the contribution of values-based practice and empowerment perspectives

- The skill base that social work brings to multidisciplinary mental health practice including communication skills; assessment, relationship-based practice; building partnerships; advocacy and utilising social work intervention methods.

The context of practice

From institution to community

Social work, perhaps more than most professions, is shaped by the context in which it is practised. Consequently, it will be helpful to review briefly the broad historical development of the pattern of mental health services. Put at its simplest, this has been a story of transition from treatment and care based in large institutions to care in the community, although that simple statement belies substantial areas of controversy, including disagreement about the main engines of reform (whether they are political and professional self-interest), what is meant by the concept of the community, and to what extent has de-institutionalisation been achieved.

The historical and sociological analysis of mental health services has undoubtedly been heavily influenced by the work of French social theorist Michel Foucault (e.g., Miller and Rose 1986; Porter 2003). His seminal work, *Madness and Civilization* (1961), argued that the template for treatment of people with mental health problems since the seventeenth century has been the treatment in the Middle Ages of people who had leprosy. This contagious disease had been introduced to Europe by soldiers and others returning from the crusades. It was contained and eventually eliminated (despite a lack of any scientific understanding of the disease) by containment of infected individuals in large institutions located away from centres of population. This approach and its efficacy, Foucault argued, became a model for the management in Western societies of social deviance, including mental illness. This accompanied a transition in attitudes in the seventeenth century brought on by the philosophical epoch known as the Enlightenment, which saw difference and non-conformity as the basis of categorising individuals as 'other' and even non-human. Thus, Foucault argues, the 'great confinement' began across Europe that involved the building of large institutions, located away from towns and cities within which were detained those who transgress against social norms, initially on an undifferentiated basis, lumping together criminals, older people, people with impairments and people with mental health problems.

Some time has been spent here outlining Foucault's argument because, although its detail is heavily disputed by other historians, it contains important perspectives for critiquing the subsequent evolution of mental health services. In the 1840s, legislation was passed in Britain requiring every county to have its own 'county asylum' for the treatment of the mentally disordered. These institutions housed, in addition to those who appeared mentally disordered, individuals who had socially transgressed including a significant number of women whose only 'sickness' was that they had been unmarried mothers. Social work was represented within these asylums as 'almoners', terminology which is in itself a legacy of the monasteries within which there were individuals responsible for the dispensation of welfare to the poor and needy. In 1974 the contracts of employment of social workers located within hospitals was transferred from the National Health Service to the newly emergent post-Seebohm local authority social services departments, although the social workers remained located within hospital settings.

By the 1960s pressure was building to dismantle this regime of institutionally based care, not least under the direction of the Conservative Minister for Health, Enoch Powell, someone not associated with progressive views. Indeed, there is disputation between historians about why the era of asylums was brought to a close. The main lines of argument divide between the so-called Whig historians who view reform as part of the process of gradual enlightenment in the approach to mental disorder of professionals and the wider public, and those of a more Marxian persuasion who saw this as part of a 'fiscal crisis' of welfare states, that they could not afford to maintain crumbling Victorian institutions (Scull 1977). Others detect the influence of the pharmaceutical companies (Rose 2007), who had begun to manufacture and market so-called 'major tranquilisers' for the treatment of psychotic conditions, which offered the prospect of maintaining people outside hospital through the use of depot (slow release) injections. For those commentators who drew on Foucault's analysis, this scenario explains how the psychiatric professions were able to maintain their medical sphere of influence even without the physical existence of the asylums, that they could consolidate their claim to expertise and extend their power and control into non-institutional settings through the use of these new drugs.

This controversy continues, but whatever the academic disputation, the empirical reality for the last twenty to thirty years has been the progressive closure of the asylums, the development of smaller units with fewer beds in locations closer to home, and the development of services in the community, many of which operate without the availability of residential beds. This trend has run in parallel with the broader development in health and social care of 'care in the community' or 'community care'. This policy development incorporates several themes but includes the philosophy that care should be available on a personalised basis reasonably close to where people live, that it should be available on the basis of people's needs rather than the interests of professionals and, controversially, that the introduction of market mechanisms would create more efficiency and responsiveness in services. These objectives were enshrined in the National Health Service and Community Care Act (1990) and, despite innumerable shifts in the detail of policy, not least the introduction of internal markets into service development, this has remained the broad direction of travel.

The development of social work within mental health services has followed, and sometimes prefigured, this transition from institution to community. The first qualified mental health social workers were employed in the UK in the 1920s with the first mental health social work training course in the United Kingdom beginning at the London School of Economics in 1929 (CSIP/NIMHE 2007). The training was influenced by psychosocial explanations of mental distress. Social workers were employed in the community in child guidance clinics as well as psychiatric hospitals. At the time, hospital-based social workers were the only professional group of mental health workers to bridge both the hospital and the community settings. Much of their work was focused on the assessment of family and social circumstances. Even in the beginnings of the profession, mental health social workers had a clear identity grounded within an explicit value base. For example, in 1939 the Association of Psychiatric Social Workers declined the suggestion from the British Medical Association to become registered as medical auxiliaries (CSIP/NIMHE 2007).

Integration of services

A further message of the community care agenda has been the assumption that services lacked coordination; that sometimes they duplicated provision, leading to what has been referred to as 'death by assessment' or alternatively gaps in the provision of services. Consequently, in parallel with the process of deinstitutionalisation has been movement towards integration of services, notably health and social care services. In mental health this has a somewhat longer history than in relation to areas such as children's or adult care services. As long ago as 1975 *Better Services for the Mentally Ill* (Department of Health and Social Security 1975) provided joint funding between the NHS and social services for new initiatives, though progress was patchy and haphazard (Fawcett and Karban 2005). Also, the Care Programme Approach (discussed in more detail below), introduced in 1991, required coordination between services. The requirement under the Care Programme Approach to appoint a 'keyworker' (later 'care coordinator') signalled in the genericism of these roles that traditional professional roles and boundaries should be superseded by roles defined by generic function.

Chapter 8

A recurrent theme of mental health policy is the characterisation of people with mental health problems as being dangerous (the fallacious nature of this assumption is discussed in Chapter 8) and this has also been a driver towards service integration. A series of public inquiries into homicides committed by people with histories of mental disorder have cited lack of service coordination as a contributory factor in these tragedies. The landmark inquiry in this respect was in relation to Christopher Clunis (Ritchie et al., 1994), an ex-patient who stabbed to death Jonathan Zito on Finsbury Park station. Clunis was someone who had led a fairly itinerant life and drifted out of contact with services.

The public climate created by these cases contributed to the view taken by the incoming Labour government in 1997 that 'community care was dead'. This did not signal a return to institutionalisation but rather a determination to drive through reorganisation of services, mainly under the rhetorical mantle of 'modernisation'. Professional roles were to become less strongly demarcated so that there was greater flexibility about who did what, and boundaries between services became more blurred so that individuals did not 'slip through the net' and received 'joined up services' (these clichés have tended to characterise this debate). The blueprint for the reconfiguration of services was developed in a series of White Papers and in particular the *National Service Framework for Mental Health* published in 1999 (Department of Health 1999). The Health Act (1999), implemented in 2000, gave statutory permission for progression of integration with the creation of so-called 'Health Act flexibilities'. These allowed NHS mental health services and councils with social services responsibilities to formalise partnerships, many of which had already begun to develop under informal arrangements. Flexibilities covered various activities including pooled budgets, delegation of commissioning and arrangements for integrated provision of services (Bogg 2008). The legislative permission created under the 1999 Act has now been superseded by Section 75 of the NHS Act (2006) but the essential nature of the flexibilities remains the same.

The implications of this for social work practice are far-reaching. Many social workers had already been working in mental health settings under a variety of secondment arrangements, but have now been caught up in processes of statutorily based service integration which some commentators have described as over-prescriptive and directive (see Glasby and Peck 2003); workers have found themselves answerable to multiple inspection and regulation regimes, and ambiguities concerning who employs them and establishing clear lines of accountability. The sites within which these tensions are primarily experienced and played out by mental health social workers are within mental health teams.

Teamwork and multidisciplinarity

Chapter 9

A deeper examination of the development within mental health services of specialist teams, and the skills of multidisciplinary work are given more extensive analysis in Chapter 9 but here, in terms of setting the scene of mental health social work, we need to consider the broad issues posed by the context of service integration and multidisciplinarity. As we have seen, it can be argued that mental health social work practice has longer antecedents of multidisciplinary teamwork than other mainstream areas of practice. Social workers in mental health teams typically find themselves located in settings where they may be the only representative of their profession. This is quite different from the position of social workers who work in adult services or children and families teams that have devolved from generic post-Seebohm social services departments, where social work represented the dominant professional ethos, often led by senior management teams who were social work trained.

Mental health social workers work in multidisciplinary teams which will typically contain psychiatrists, clinical psychologists, community psychiatric nurses (CPNs) and perhaps others such as occupational therapists, development workers and support workers. This environment brings opportunities and challenges. For some social workers this is part of the attraction of mental health practice, that it brings the intellectual stimulation of working alongside others who bring alternative perspectives and methods. However, a significant amount of research also shows that mental health workers have to cope with a range of tensions. These have been usefully summarised by Bogg (2008). There is *role ambiguity and conflict,* where there are boundary disputes about whose responsibility it is to undertake particular duties, perhaps offering information on statutory rights, or providing particular psychosocial interventions such as family therapy. This can lead to very basic professional insecurities about the validity of the contribution made by a team member. *Communication difficulties* can arise where team members have been educated and socialised within the particular frameworks of their profession, be it the psychological theories underpinning the clinical psychologist's training, the medical orientation of the psychiatrist, or the values-based orientation of social work training. Such differences manifest themselves through the discourse of the team, and even very basic discussions about whether people with mental health problems should be referred to as patients, service users or clients. Communication difficulties are also often compounded by incompatibility of information systems, where health and social care databases are developed and owned separately. The *development of a team ethos* or shared identity can be hampered by these competing professional orientations and rivalries. The strong possibility that individuals will be line managed by someone from a different professional background, overlain perhaps by dual lines of accountability to management and clinical structures, exacerbates these tensions and can produce *lack of faith in management understanding and effectiveness*. The *hierarchical* nature of health and social care organisation and the experience of being line managed by another profession can produce overt or covert *power* struggles, not least where an occupational group such as social workers feel that a social perspective is inherently threatened by the status and dominance of clinical professionals. Finally, all of this can generate *priority and perspective conflicts*, where each professional believes that their own approach justifies setting priorities for service users or service developments that are disputed by others, perhaps a social worker feels that their commitment to developing social inclusion initiatives is undermined by a team focus on monitoring compliance with pharmacological treatment.

It may be felt that all this overemphasises the negative aspects of multidisciplinary working and neglects the potential benefits of service users receiving whole person care. However, it is important to note that this cumulative evidence from research into integration has to be acknowledged if the dysfunctional aspects of multidisciplinary teamwork are to be addressed and overcome. This has been the subject of various government and voluntary sector initiatives, not least the Department of Health's 'capable practitioner' initiative and New Ways of Working programme. These have addressed the challenges of multidisciplinary work by seeking to identify the core competencies that should be part of any practitioner's toolkit, whatever their professional identity ('The Ten Essential Shared Capabilities',

Chapter 9

considered in detail in Chapter 9), and the specific and distinct contributions that can be made by the various professions within the mental health arena (the New Ways of Working programme, see CSIP/NIMHE 2007). Thus, it is hoped to support practitioners by emphasising their commonalities whilst also defining their particular expertise.

Care management and the Care Programme Approach

A key role in the introduction of community care in adult services was the creation of the role of the care manager. This was the person who was responsible for assessing the service users' needs for services and then was responsible for creating a 'package of care', a collection of services that met the needs that had been identified. Influential research by the Personal Social Services Research Unit (PSSRU) had evaluated 'case management', the forerunner from the United States of care management, as a more efficient and effective method of delivering services to older people with complex needs than traditional models of service delivery (Challis et al., 1990). It is a matter of contention whether the PSSRU evidence was appropriately generalised as the template for the new approach to service delivery, but this was the approach embraced by the Department of Health for community care implementation. Social workers were drafted in to be redesignated as care managers; some felt that they had become bureaucratic functionaries who had been forced to renounce their traditional therapeutic role, others claimed they could subvert the care management process to retain their 'true' social work identity (Baldwin 2000) and some embraced care management as a method that allowed social workers to combine creatively their former role with new, innovative responsibilities for commissioning services (Gilbert 2003).

Within mental health services, case management took a different path to implementation. Contemporaneous with the introduction of care management, but also influenced by the moral panic surrounding the Christopher Clunis case, discussed earlier, and the Spokes case (a service user who killed social worker Isabel Schwartz (Schneider 1993, cited Pritchard 2006)), the Care Programme Approach (CPA) was introduced in 1991 as a mental health variant of care management (Department of Health 1991). As is suggested by this allusion to a high-profile homicide case, in the mental health arena the assessment of need was hitched to the assessment of the risk of the service user to others. It was followed in 1994 by the creation of Supervision Registers in order to monitor the supervision of high-risk service users. CPA in its original guise contained four elements:

- The assessment of health and social needs for those referred to specialist mental health services.

- The drawing up by the clinical team of a care plan which identified who was to deliver the various elements of the care package.

- Appointment of a key worker (later redesignated as a care coordinator) to monitor and coordinate the elements of the care package.

- Regular review and adaptation of the care plan.

CPA indicated a commitment to multidisciplinarity with the non-specification of the professional background of the key worker who could be any individual within the team, usually a social worker, nurse or occupational therapist. A plan is formulated at a team meeting, usually attended by the service user and carers. The agenda of the meeting will be to specify the context of the service user's problems, assess their personal circumstances, identify their medical, psychological and social needs, and draw up a care plan to address these needs. Until an official review in 2008 (Department of Health 2008a) of the care planning system, anyone could be the subject of CPA, although there were two levels of intensity of the approach, depending on whether individuals presented ordinary or enhanced levels of need, usually more narrowly interpreted as risk. CPA has been the subject of dissatisfaction by professionals and service users alike (and has never been implemented in Wales). Although at a policy level CPA seemed benign and balanced in its approach, at the local implementation mental health workers often claimed it was a formalistic and bureaucratic exercise that required boxes to be ticked but constrained the exercise of professional judgement (Rogers and Pilgrim 2001). Surveys of service users revealed confusion, often individuals did not know whether or not they were subject to CPA, or even who their care coordinator was and they complained that the contents of assessments were not shared with them (Rose 2001).

There has been extensive consultation over the delivery of CPA, and the Department of Health has reformed the system in an attempt to 'refocus' the approach (Department of Health 2007c; Department of Health 2008b)). Part of the reconstruction of the policy is an emphasis on CPA as a cornerstone of the 'personalisation agenda', that is, the espoused shift towards maximising service choice and individualising the match between need and services. The two levels of CPA have been abandoned, with just one level, equivalent to enhanced level, for all people who have been subject to detention under the 1983 Mental Health Act. Individuals subject to CPA will have available to them:

- support from a care coordinator;
- a comprehensive multidisciplinary and multi-agency assessment of needs;
- an assessment of financial needs including direct payments (see below);
- a written comprehensive care plan including risk and contingency plans;
- assessment of needs for advocacy services;
- periodic review of the care plan;
- information given to carers of their entitlement to assessment of their needs.

At the policy level the new CPA approach is justified in terms of the personalisation agenda, but the reality is that it is restricted to those individuals who have been subject to compulsion. The argument for this refocusing is a more targeted use of scarce resources, but it can also be seen as rationing comprehensive assessment to a relatively small number of service users, with the danger that CPA will be stigmatising in its effect by its association with compulsory powers. Social workers will find themselves continuing to be designated as care coordinators where they are the most appropriate person to work with a given individual, but may be dependent on all their skills to make CPA a positive experience for the service user.

Personalisation and direct payments

As we have seen, there have been themes which have been consistently developing through both Conservative and Labour administrations in relation to deinstitutionalisation, diversification of suppliers of care through the introduction of market mechanisms and the promotion of 'choice'. At times it seems that many policy initiatives are introduced as reforms of mainstream healthcare delivery, and mental health is an afterthought. How the headline reforms are to be interpreted and implemented to be meaningful in mental health contexts is often devolved to 'modernisation' agencies such as the National Institute for Mental Health England (NIMHE).

An umbrella term that has been emerging for aspects of reform has been the concept of 'personalisation', a later manifestation of the so-called 'choice agenda'. The Green Paper *Independence,*

Well-being and Choice (Department of Health 2005) set out the terms of reference for this vision, and were then amplified in the White Paper *Our Health, Our Care, Our Say: A new direction for community services* (Department of Health 2006a). The core messages of these policies are expressed in the executive summary:

> This White Paper confirms the vision in the Green Paper of high-quality support meeting people's aspirations for independence and greater control over their lives, making services flexible and responsive to individual needs.

One of the main mechanisms for extending the notion of choice and control has been through direct payments. Direct payments are a means by which people who require social care directly receive community care monies so that they can choose and pay for their own support to meet their needs. Local authorities have a duty to offer direct payments to those assessed as eligible but take-up of direct payments has been slow and variable within mental health, with some commentators finding a correlation between low levels of implementation, and local authorities with protectionist attitudes towards public sector jobs (Riddell et al., 2005). A study of direct payments for users of mental health services in Scotland concluded that a significant obstacle to implementation was the low level of awareness amongst professionals of the potential of the scheme, and lack of flexibility in devising innovative approaches to supporting independence (Ridley and Jones 2003). A research study by the Joseph Rowntree Foundation sought to identify factors that would make a difference to take-up of direct payments by mental health service users (Newbigging with Lowe 2005) and these are summarised in Box 3.1.

Box 3.1   Factors that could make a difference to take-up of direct payments by mental health service users

- Service users, carers and professionals require straightforward, accurate and accessible information about direct payments which is specific to mental health.

- Both service users and professionals can be confused about the distinction to access to an assessment for receipt of direct payments and access to services, where the threshold may be much higher and based largely on clinical considerations. This can affect take-up.

- Mental health users require specific advocacy and practical support to facilitate access to and use of direct payments.

- The absence of a streamlined process integrated with the Care Programme Approach adds to the sense of direct payments being a burden rather than an opportunity.

- Ways to increase take-up by people from black and minority ethnic communities include developing resources and approaches, including outreach and direct support services specific to those communities.

- A change in the culture of mental health service provision is required. This would need a tangible commitment to promoting self-determination, evident in the way staff interact and support people experiencing mental distress.

- Introducing direct payments requires effective leadership to drive the process of implementation from national direction and guidance through to local leadership, at both a strategic and an operational level.

- Fostering partnerships across organisations and supporting collaborative problem-solving could facilitate learning about the implementation of direct payments.

- Introducing direct payments in a planned way requires thought as to how existing services can be reviewed, reconfigured and recommissioned.

- There is a need to review what direct payments cover in mental health: the distinction between health and social care in mental health is not an easy one, and arguably no longer relevant given the integration of health and social care to provide mental health services.

(Newbigging with Lowe 2005: x–xi)

The personalisation agenda is not without critics, some of whom claim that the term is used in inconsistent and contradictory ways (Cutler et al., 2007). Ferguson has argued that the development of these approaches is part of a move to shift risk from the state to the individual, and that 'the philosophy of personalisation is not one that social workers should accept uncritically' (Ferguson 2007: 387).

The social work role in 'new' mental health services

Chapter 9

The evolving 'modernisation' of mental health services towards care in the community, integration of services and multidisciplinarity has generated for the various professions uncertainty about their role and identity. This has been formally addressed through a government-sponsored programme of work led by NIMHE called New Ways of Working (CSIP/ NIMHE 2007), also discussed in Chapter 9. A series of special interest groups and working parties, including one for social work, sought to articulate the distinct but complementary contribution of each profession. The report confirmed that social work values, skills and knowledge already encompass the approaches set out in current government policy which have already been indicated, including the

Mental Health Bill, the Green Paper *Independence, Well-being and Choice* and the social inclusion agenda. All emphasise the need for service users to participate actively in their own care. Social workers have historically worked in partnership with service users to which, more than any other profession, their value base is most closely aligned. As the report states, 'Social work is therefore a crucial component to mental health service development if stated policy objectives are to be achieved' (CSIP/NIMHE 2007). The New Ways of Working programme endorses the centrality of social work to mental health services in ways that most social workers probably welcome, although the value base needs to be further elaborated and critiqued.

Values-based practice

Social work tends to struggle to define its contribution to the caring professions in terms of its methods or knowledge base: methods tend to be common with other disciplines such as psychology – for example, cognitive behavioural approaches – and its knowledge-base draws widely from the social sciences. Instead, it is sometimes argued that social work is values-based and it is those values that make social work distinct. In relation to mental health practice these assertions about social work should not be accepted uncritically. In the context we have been considering of multidisciplinary practice, social work's knowledge base is distinct in that it is the only profession whose professional curriculum includes sociology and social policy, providing practitioners with a more structural appreciation of the nature of social problems. Social workers also have studied areas of law that impact on practice, so bring to the team context knowledge of crucial areas such as child protection. On the other hand, the other professions that are represented in mental health services would regard it as impertinent for social work to assert that it is the only profession that was mindful of and shaped by, values and principles!

Nevertheless, the discussion of values in social work has taken some distinct turns, particularly in relation to anti-discriminatory and anti-oppressive practice, when compared to the clinical disciplines. This is again quite distinct from social work's earlier discourses around values and ethics. Social work has been heavily influenced by the work of German seventeenth-century philosopher Immanuel Kant and his concept of the *categorical imperative*, namely, that we should do to other people what – in the same circumstances – we would want them to do to ourselves, and that this will hold to be universally true. The strongest legacy of Kant's ideas is in the writing of Biestek (1961) who formulates a set of universal principles of social work that would be presumed to hold true in all circumstances. Kantian thinking is also reflected in the codes of ethics that have emerged for social work in various countries, and in the UK most specifically in the General Social Care Council's (GSCC's) codes of practice. Yet, these Kantian perspectives have been strongly challenged and the critiques have particular relevance for mental health practice. The arguments of Kantians such as Biestek are premised on a principle of self-determination by individuals as to their choices and preferences. However, the underlying – often hidden – assumptions of this argument are that self-determination is only achievable by individuals with the capacity to be rational and autonomous. This seems to preclude many of the individuals who use mental health services, who the wider society would not see as being rational, having capacity to make their own choices and achieve self-determination. These traditional approaches to social work ethics appear to leave practice with people with mental health problems as vulnerable to coercive and paternalistic practice, in their 'own best interests'.

The alternative approach to ethical practice is that which is referred to as *utilitarianism*, derived from nineteenth-century philosophers such as John Stuart Mills, which rejects the individualism of Kantian ethics, and states that what is good is that which promotes the happiness of the greatest number of people. This refutes the idea of universality, that a particular action such as maintaining confidentiality will be good in all situations, and asserts that we should consider the consequences of actions – will the impact of doing this produce happiness for more people than if we did something else? Within the mental health context this again may be problematic as it may be used to justify coercive approaches to social control, restricting the liberties of people with a mental health problem, on the (usually unfounded) grounds that this is for the good of the wider society.

However, there has been a rediscovery of utilitarianism in relation to mental health policy and practice from the direction of economists, notably in the work of Richard Layard (it is no coincidence that the early utilitarians were political economists). This argument recognises that the problems of mental disorder, particularly the common disorders such as depression and anxiety, impose a heavy financial burden on society, as well as the misery of the affected individuals and their families. Layard (2005) has argued for major programmes of investment in treatments that are effective for anxiety and depression to alleviate the unhappiness of individuals, but also justified by the wider economic effi-ciencies that will be produced. This argument has been very influential with the post-1997 Labour government, giving rise to significant investment in increasing the availability of evidence-based therapies for common mental disorders. The downside to this may be that making economic utility the criterion for providing intervention may create an 'underclass' within mental health service users, people who have longer term, seemingly intractable mental health problems, who have little chance of avoiding unemployment and dependency on welfare benefits (Gould 2006a).

The very different assumptions that underpin Kantian and utilitarian approaches sometimes appear to produce irreconcilable perspectives over what should be done in a particular situation; for example, in mental health this may be in relation to different perspectives between service users (expecting to be treated as autonomous and self-determining) and families (claiming that their interests come first and that they are greater in number). Within health and social care this has stimulated interest in alter-native ethical perspectives of which two should be mentioned here. The first is a return to the writing of Aristotle, the Greek philosopher of ancient times, who emphasised the importance of considering the virtues of the person who aspires to be a good practitioner. This approach to *virtue ethics*, par-ticularly identified in social work with the American author Rhodes (1986), says that our primary concern should be to identify the traits that characterise a person that we would consider to be virtuous and how they would act to demonstrate those virtues in a given situation of dilemma. In relation to mental health practice this might direct us to think about how as practitioners we can demonstrate such virtues as compassion, courage and authenticity in decision-making. Critics of virtue ethics find such a list rather arbitrary and reflective of prevailing ideological views of the virtuous person that may derive from dominant, prejudicial attitudes.

Another important perspective that is contemporary with the revived interest in Aristotle, derives from feminist perspectives and is referred to as the *ethics of care*. Social work has tended to borrow from writing about nursing ethics in this regard, and particularly the work of Caroline Gilligan (1982). This approach claims that from the Enlightenment onwards ethical discourse has privileged values that are inherently masculine and paternalistic, espousing ideals of rugged male individualism, and has over-looked qualities that are most often demonstrated by women, which are shown through relationships with other people, particularly those that are nurturing and caring. This point of view does seem to share some terrain with virtue ethics, namely, that the determination of what is good derives from the quality demonstrated by the person, though it 'reclaims' what it means to be virtuous in terms that are asserted to be inherently feminine. Again, there are critics of this position who argue that the ethics of care are too vague to offer prescriptions for practice in particular situations, and that the premise that 'care' is always something that is good is largely unexamined (Allmark 2002). Nevertheless, feminist perspectives in relation to value positions taken by practitioners sensitise us to the inherent patriarchy of caring institutions, most dramatically revealed by surveys of abuse of women by staff and fellow-patients in mental health units.

Activity 3.1 Ethical perspectives in mental health practice

Joyce is a 33-year-old woman from a white British background who lives with her parents and 25-year-old brother, David. Three years ago Joyce was diagnosed with schizophrenia and has not worked since that time. She refuses to take medication as she says this makes her feel unwell and causes her to gain weight. She has a number of paranoid delusions that incorporate her parents and as a result she is often hostile towards them. This is causing anxiety within the family, particularly as Joyce's father has deteriorating physical health due to a heart condition. David also finds the atmosphere in the house stressful and recently asked his GP for help with feelings of depression and anxiety. Joyce's mother has recently given up her own job to stay at home because of the needs of the family were so acute. You are the social worker from the community mental health team and have been trying to discuss with Joyce other possible accommodation options, but Joyce is insistent that this is her home and she has a right to remain where she is.

Analyse this situation from Utilitarian, Kantian, virtue ethics and feminist approaches and compare and contrast the issues that are highlighted by each perspective.

Social work brings to the multidisciplinary 'table' sensitivities that are shaped by these mainstream approaches to ethics and values. Arguably though, social work's more radical and distinctive contribution derives from the broader sphere of anti-discriminatory and anti-oppressive practice. We have already commented on the structural analysis of social problems that derive from sociological understandings of mental health. This includes appreciation of the hierarchical relationships of power that exist between social groups, including the relative disadvantage of people who are mental health service users, and the over-representation within the population of mental health service users of social groups that are relatively disadvantaged, such as members of black and minority ethnic groups. Anti-discrimination and anti-oppression can also address the issues raised by feminist ethics of care, where the specific disadvantages of women within the mental health system are addressed. There is now an extensive literature in social work on these approaches, including the central contribution of Thompson (2000) through his PCS (Personal, Cultural and Social) model of anti-discriminatory practice. Thompson's argument is that progressive values need to be incorporated in practice that addresses personal, cultural and social levels. This analytical approach is generically stated, but is also an important contribution to multidisciplinary practice in mental health, and one which social workers can value as their contribution. One of the foremost psychiatrists writing about racism in mental health practice, Fernando (1991), has referred to social work as the leading discipline in this area. The influence of social work is discernible in frameworks for generic core competence in new mental health services, particularly the Ten Core Competences, as already cited.

Empowering service users and promoting autonomy

The social work literature makes extensive reference to the desirability of empowering service users and promoting their autonomy. There is a sense in which these are 'hurrah' terms, for what reasonable person could be against them, but with little analytical precision. Parsloe expressed her reservations in trenchant terms:

> It (empowerment) is a most unfortunate word for social work to have adopted because it can well be argued that the very idea that one person, a social worker, can empower another, a client, runs counter to the whole idea of greater equality of power on which the concept supposedly depends.
> (Parsloe, cited Barnes and Bowl 2001: 19)

This is sometimes referred to as the 'empowerment paradox'. Nevertheless, there have been some attempts to gain some precision in the use of these terms in order to make them meaningful aims for social intervention. Indeed, attempting to increase an individual's autonomy, their capacity to take responsibility for their lives, seems a basic aspiration of mental health social work and one which touches on fundamental human rights, and is closely linked to what we understand by 'empowerment'. Barnes and Bowl expressed this idea directly:

> If, by definition, someone experiencing severe psychological distress is perceived as having impaired autonomy then this has important implications for their level of empowerment, both because of the impact this can have on perceptions of self, and because this can lead to actions which reduce objective opportunities to exercise autonomy.
> (Barnes and Bowl 2001: 8–9)

In a very influential theoretical examination of the concept of autonomy, Doyal and Gough (1991) argue that this is a basic and universal human need, one that will be shaped by local cultural norms, but fundamental to the well-being of all people. Their arguments for universal definitions of need are supported by international empirical evidence that they support well-being. They identify the factors that are necessary to achieve autonomy, regardless of cultural context, and it is useful to set these out as criteria for considering whether social work intervention is indeed supportive of the enlargement of a person's autonomy. These are:

- having the capacity to formulate aims and beliefs common to a form of life;
- having confidence to want to act and to participate in a form of life;
- being able to participate socially, formulating aims and beliefs and the ability to communicate with others about them;
- being able to understand that actions have been done by them and not by someone else;
- being able to understand the external, objective constraints on one's actions;
- being able to take responsibility for what one does.

Sometimes users of mental health services are judged (and condemned) on the basis of whether they possess 'insight'. This is a slippery concept with no fixed meaning within psychiatry, but can be little more than the judgement of a professional about whether their definition of a situation is accepted by the service user (i.e., if they do not, then they lack insight). Unpacking, in the way exemplified by Doyal and Gough, the ingredients of the concept of autonomy may well be a more empirically grounded approach to thinking about what needs to be achieved in order to live a life that is self-determined but also socially engaged.

Skills for practice

Functioning effectively within the context as discussed in this chapter requires social workers to be skilful as well as knowledgeable. Within subsequent chapters dealing with particular kinds of mental health problem, we will consider specific methods and skills relevant to those problems. However, mental health social work builds on many of the generic skills that are fundamental to contemporary social work practice. They are covered in detail in generalist textbooks but here we touch on some aspects that are particularly relevant to mental health.

Communication

The 1983 Mental Health Act requires that service users are interviewed 'in a suitable manner'. Although this stricture specifically relates to assessments for compulsory admissions to hospital, it is a principle that should underpin all mental health practice. The intention of the Act was not only that individuals should be seen face to face, but that the interviewer should be culturally competent and proactive in anticipating and meeting the needs someone may have that require special help in order to communicate. This may include interviewing someone who is not sufficiently proficient in the English language. Assessing someone's mental state requires attention to the nuances of language, particularly if metaphorical expression is not to be mistaken for a delusional belief. An interpreter may be needed, and there should be sensitivity to the possibility that a family member will probably not be appropriate, or possibly a member of the interviewee's local community, where matters of confidentiality or norms of cultural appropriateness may be jeopardised. It should be remembered that people with hearing impairments are disproportionately represented amongst people with mental health problems, and an interpreter with signing skills might need to be called upon (Ridgeway 1997).

Communicating with individuals with delusional beliefs also requires tact and skill: directly challenging a belief may provoke irritability or even aggression, while collusion (unquestioning agreement) can be condescending as well as reinforcing the delusion. A neutral position needs to be maintained where the social worker indicates that she is hearing what is being expressed, and acknowledges the emotion accompanying what is being said such as anger or fear, but without literal acceptance of the delusion. Where the person is withdrawn and even mute, a social worker needs to have the capacity to show that they can be alongside someone and accept their feelings, even though nothing is being directly communicated other than through body language. If someone has a condition that involves impairment of short-term memory, patience is required to repeat information, or to use additional devices to make sure that something is remembered, for instance putting important information in writing.

Assessment

Assessment is perhaps the most important stage in the care management process, and it is also central to the care plan approach. However, as has been discussed, there is also social worker dissatisfaction with the extent to which assessment has become proceduralised with tightly proscribed items to be completed and entitlements to be quantified. Yet psychosocial assessment is a rich part of the heritage of social work's legacy, particularly within mental health practice where social histories have traditionally made a fundamental contribution to holistic psychiatric assessments. A person's early history, the dynamics of their family, their experiences of living and working within their community offers profound insights into the nature of a person's problems and psychological distress. Similarly, the variation of someone's condition may reflect anniversaries of significant events in the person's earlier life, or a social history may uncover patterns in the onset of a person's distress, revealing the triggers for changes in their mental health. All this makes a strong case for the continuation of social workers bringing their assessment skills to multidisciplinary team working. At the same time there has to be sensitivity to over-intrusion into the lives of people who may be in contact with several agencies and service users, and carers alike are rightly upset when assessment becomes repetitive and intrusive.

Working through relationships

A theme that repeatedly emerges from debates about care management and care planning has been the anxiety that these approaches replace social work's emphasis on the importance of establishing productive relationships with users of services with bureaucratic and impersonal procedures. Recent years has seen the 'rediscovery' of the relationship as a primary element of practice through which effective practice can be delivered. This is being referred to as relationship-based practice (Ruch 2005) and connects directly with early social work traditions of psychosocial practice, informed by concerns with the inner, emotional world of the individual along with external social factors. Wilson et al. (2008) have identified the core elements of relationship-based practice as: acceptance of the uniqueness of any encounter between social worker and service user; recognition of the complex interplay of conscious and unconscious motivations influencing behaviour; the importance of psychosocial responses to problems; recognition that the relationship is an element of any intervention; and it stresses the 'use of self' and relationship as the medium through which an intervention is delivered. In mental health practice, the social worker's success in making a relationship may be severely challenged when a service user at times of distress presents behaviour that breaches social norms; this may include unusual levels of suspicion, fear, withdrawal and emotional volatility. Patience and persistence are premium virtues. Although their research was undertaken some years ago, the findings of Truax and Carkhuff (1967) remain pertinent, that the most effective relationships for achieving therapeutic success demonstrate unconditional positive regard for the other person, empathy with their feelings and congruence.

Advocacy

Modern welfare systems comprising networks of services, each with their own criteria of entitlement for services, are characterised by complexity. Many people who wish to access services or who feel they are without control of circumstances that effect their lives are possibly going to seek advocacy to establish their entitlement or autonomy. The role of social work may be to advocate on someone's behalf, to support them to advocate on their own behalf, or to refer them to a specialist advocacy agency. Both the Mental Capacity Act 2005 and Mental Health Act 2007 now provide for specialist advocacy support for individuals in defined circumstances. Some of the considerations that applied to communication carried across to advocacy. Members of some black and minority ethnic groups find themselves over-represented in the population of people with mental health problems, and yet under-represented amongst the people able to obtain supportive services. They may also have special advocacy needs in terms of understanding of their cultural and socioeconomic situation (Rai-Atkins et al., 2002). Research shows that specialist advocacy services are thin on the ground (Atkinson 1999), and that there are particular gaps in relation to groups most disadvantaged by mental health services such as African–Caribbean men (Newbigging et al., 2007). Bateman (1995) identifies the core skills of advocacy as: interviewing – being able to elicit what the service user wants and any relevant information; being able to be assertive in presenting a case without slipping into being aggressive; skills of negotiation; self-management (making use of yourself as a resource); research skills to find and collate information and 'litigation' skills (being able to present a case cogently to an arbitrator).

Building partnerships

It has become something of a truism to argue that the full complexity of people's lives cannot be addressed by one agency, and that the assembly of packages of care requires practitioners to be able to work alongside and in cooperation with workers from other agencies. 'Partnership' has come to be an all-embracing term applied to collaboration at so many levels that it may have lost terminological exactitude. Despite this, mental health social workers find themselves working within organisations that describe themselves as 'partnership trusts' by virtue of the various forms of combination of health and social care services. The normative presumption is that partnerships produce better outcomes for service users but the research evidence for this is inconclusive (Glasby and Dickinson 2008). Interestingly for the purposes of this volume, one of the most significant case studies of partnership working is of a mental health service, the Somerset Partnership NHS and Social Care Trust (Peck et al., 2002). A significant finding was that the process of coming together produced a 'J'-curve effect, where the organisation experienced short-term decline in morale and efficiency before improvement began to be experienced. The lesson seems to be that workers should not expect immediate improvement. At the same time, and this is part of the ambiguity of the evidence-base, surveys of service users also found mixed results with better service coordination but concerns about reductions in therapeutic support. Despite these inconclusive messages from research, social workers will de facto for the foreseeable future find themselves working within partnership organisations. Glasby and Dickinson (2008) have attempted to distil the messages from research for practice in partnerships and identify as the primary lessons the need to clarify terminology so that the objectives of a partnership are understood, to make identification of desired outcomes the priority around which specific partnership relationships are formed and not to assume automatically that partnership is the best approach to a given problem.

Using social work intervention methods

Social work is often in thrall to the methods of other professional disciplines, particularly clinical psychology, but should not overlook that it has its own 'indigenous' methods of intervention which are evidence-based and applicable in working with people with mental health problems. It is beyond the scope of this book to review the totality of social work methods but there are compendiums available to students and practitioners such as Payne's *Modern Social Work Theory* (2005). An example would be task-centred practice, a structured and time-limited approach that was developed entirely within social work (Reid and Shyne 1969; Reid and Epstein 1972; Kirk and Reid 2002). Subsequent research has shown this to be effective with a range of moderately complex service user problems (Reid 1978; Goldberg 1985).

Key points

- The main historical shift in the delivery of mental health services has been from hospital-based care to care in the community, though concerns remain that these non-institutional services can still create dependency and impede recovery.

- Social workers in mental health settings have had to adapt to working in multidisciplinary teams, though the advantages and disadvantages of integration are still not fully evaluated. In mental health services, care management has been delivered through the Care Programme Approach. There are concerns that the system is increasingly used to justify rationing services to a small number of service users who are deemed to be high risk.

- The current policy agenda emphasises personalisation but the implications for implementing this in mental health practice are contested.

- Social work brings to multidisciplinary teamwork a values-based approach that is strongly grounded in anti-discriminatory and anti-oppressive approaches to practice.

- Social work theory and methods also contribute to the skills mix of multidisciplinary teamwork through their communication, relationship, assessment, advocacy, partnership-building and intervention skills.

Key reading

Barnes, M. and Bowl, R. (2001) *Taking Over The Asylum: Empowerment and Mental Health*, Basingstoke: Palgrave.

Bogg, D. (2008) *The Integration of Mental Health Social Work and the NHS*, Exeter: Learning Matters.

Carr, S. (2008) *SCIE Report 20: Personalisation: A Rough Guide*, London: Social Care Institute for Excellence. Online. Available online: http://www.scie.org.uk/publications/reports/report20.pdf (accessed 12 May 2009).

4 Working with children and adolescents

By the end of this chapter you should have an understanding of:

- The prevalence of mental health problems in children and the development of services to meet their needs

- The policy context of services for children with mental health problems, including the National Service Framework

- Types of behaviour disorders in children, including conduct disorders, oppositional defiant disorder and attention deficit hyperactivity disorder

- Developmental disorders, including autism and Asperger's syndrome

- Emotional disorders in children, including childhood depression, enuresis, encopresis and elective or selective mutism

- Approaches to working with parents who have mental health problems

- The need to coordinate mental health services for children and adults.

Introduction – the policy and practice context

Although there are differing theoretical explanations of why childhood mental health and psychological well-being are so important for later life, there is at this time better knowledge about the prevalence and incidence of children's mental health problems in the UK than ever before, not least because of the Office for National Statistics community-based survey (Meltzer et al., 2000; Green et al., 2004). Ten per cent of 5 to 15 year olds have a diagnosable mental health disorder, which if extrapolated to the population of England and Wales, means that around 1.1 million children and young people could benefit from specialist help. Of that number, up to 45,000 have a severe mental health problem. Although the surveys estimate the magnitude of the problems, they also make it clear that many of these children and young people – around 40 per cent – are not in contact with relevant services. There is a danger that social workers located in mainstream settings will regard children and young people's mental health as a specialist area which can be left to the experts. Surveys and studies of 'caseness' in referrals to services (e.g., Huxley et al., 1987) show that *all* social workers need to have some understanding and recognition of children's mental health problems, when to refer for specialist help, and when to reassure families that some 'problems' are within the range of normal child development.

Not least among the reasons why social workers should be concerned with children and young people's mental health problems are that many of them are associated with adverse social factors leading to social exclusion. Mental disorders are more common in older than younger children: in 2004, 10 per cent of boys and 5 per cent of girls aged 5–10 were found to have a disorder compared with 13 per cent and 10 per cent of those aged 11–16 (Meltzer et al., 2000). As with other measures of disadvantage, boys overall have worse mental health than girls. Children and young people who live in families with a low household income or with no parent working or in families with a lone parent are also more prone to have a diagnosable mental disorder. As with any interpretation of data, it should be remembered that these are correlations – statistical associations – and cannot be assumed to be causal. A recent report into the working of Child and Adolescent Mental Health Services (Department of Health 2006b) reminds us that the majority of children and young people in these circumstances grow and develop without difficulties. Just as there are correlations with family factors, there are also associations with educational attainment, absences from school, school exclusions, strength of friendship networks, physical health and offending behaviour (CAMHS Review 2008).

Some children in special circumstances have greater needs regarding their mental health. The following statistics are reported in the *National Service Framework for Children, Young People and Maternity Services* (Department of Health 2004b): looked after children are five times more likely than their peers to have a mental health disorder; children and young people with significant learning disabilities are three to four times more likely to have a mental disorder and at least 40 per cent of young offenders have been found to have a diagnosable mental health disorder.

Despite the prevalence of the problems, services have developed in an ad hoc and patchy manner. Mental health services for children and young people are conventionally described as belonging to four tiers of service, grouped in increasing levels of specialisation from community-based health promotion to acute treatment services (Department of Health 2004b):

- Tier 1: Primary care services including GPs, paediatricians, health visitors, school nurses, social workers, teachers, juvenile justice workers, voluntary agencies and social services.

- Tier 2: CAMH services provided by professionals relating to workers in primary care including clinical child psychologists, paediatricians with specialist training in mental health, educational psychologists, child and adolescent psychiatrists, child and adolescent psychotherapists, counsellors, community nurses/nurse specialists and family therapists.

- Tier 3: CAMH specialised services for more severe, complex or persistent disorders including child and adolescent psychiatrists, clinical child psychologists, nurses (community or inpatient), child and adolescent psychotherapists, occupational therapists, speech and language therapists, art, music and drama therapists, and family therapists.

- Tier 4: CAMH tertiary-level services such as day units, highly specialised outpatient teams and inpatient units.

There are some grounds for believing that children and young people's mental health has been moving up the policy agenda. The *National Framework for Children, Young People and Maternity Services* was published in 2004 (Department of Health 2004b), of which standard 9 is a chapter devoted to the mental health and psychological well-being of children and young people. The National Framework attempts to establish frameworks for practice which are evidence-based, and sets out ten markers for successful services, which are summarised in Box 4.1. It is intended that the Framework should also work to the same ends as *Every Child Matters* (Department of Children, Schools and Families 2004), reflecting underpinning principles of prevention and early intervention through integrated services.

Box 4.1 **The *National Service Framework for Children, Young People and Maternity Services* ten markers for successful services**

- All staff working directly with children and young people have sufficient knowledge, training and support to promote the psychological well-being of children, young people and their families and to identify early indicators of difficulty.

- Protocols for referral, support and early intervention are agreed between all agencies.

- Child and adolescent mental health (CAMH) professionals provide a balance of direct and indirect services and are flexible about where children, young people and families are seen in order to improve access to high levels of CAMH expertise.

- Children and young people are able to receive urgent mental health care when required, leading to a specialist mental health assessment where necessary within 24 hours or the next working day.

- Child and adolescent mental health services are able to meet the needs of all young people including those aged 16 and 17.

- All children and young people with both a learning disability and a mental health disorder have access to appropriate child and adolescent mental health services.

- The needs of children and young people with complex, severe and persistent behavioural and mental health needs are met through a multi-agency approach. Contingency arrangements are agreed at senior officer levels between health, social services and education to meet the needs and manage the risks associated with this particular group.

- Arrangements are in place to ensure that specialist multidisciplinary teams are of sufficient size and have an appropriate skill-mix, training and support to function effectively.

- Children and young people who require admission to hospital for mental health care have access to appropriate care in an environment suited to their age and development.

- When children and young people are discharged from inpatient services into the community and when young people are transferred from child to adult services, their continuity of care is ensured by use of the 'care programme approach'.

(Department of Health 2004b)

The transformation of services for children and young people will not be achieved only through improvement of specialist CAMH services; there are implications for a broad range of policies and programmes. Relevant initiatives include Sure Start, Children's Centres, Extended Schools and programmes to improve behaviour and the social and emotional aspects of learning within schools (SEAL) and the Healthy Schools Programme. This proliferation of initiatives brings considerable problems of coordination and the challenges are considerable. It is not only the institutional arrangements and lines of responsibility that are unclear, there is a blurred relationship between the various assessment systems that are contained in policy and legislation; for example, the Common Assessment

Framework, Special Educational Needs, Youth Justice, Children in Need and the Care Programme Approach. This can lead to the impression that more effort is being expended on repeated assessment than working with the child, young person and their family to address needs (CAMHS Review 2008).

Social workers, whether working in specialist CAMHS settings or in other services that address the needs of children should have a basic understanding of the main categories of disorders in children, and forms of intervention that are indicated by current research. These can be categorised as behaviour disorders, developmental disorders and emotional disorders.

Behaviour disorders

Conduct disorders

Conduct disorders constitute the largest single group of psychiatric disorders in children and adolescents and are the main reason for referral to child and adolescent mental health services (Green et al., 2004). They are characterised by a repetitive and persistent pattern of antisocial, aggressive or defiant conduct. Sociological critics of psychiatric diagnostic categories sometimes argue that conduct disorders are no more than 'dustbin' categories for antisocial behaviour, but it needs to be appreciated that conduct disorder is more severe and sustained than ordinary childish mischief or adolescent rebelliousness, and goes beyond isolated antisocial acts. To meet the Diagnostic and Statistical Manual, fourth edition (*DSM-IV*) and the International Classification of Diseases, tenth edition (*ICD-10*) definitions of conduct disorder, at least three behavioural criteria (including aggression to people and/or animals, destruction of property, deceitfulness, or theft and serious violation of rules) have to have been exhibited in the preceding twelve months, with at least one criterion present in the last six months (American Psychiatric Association 1994; World Health Organization 1992).

Conduct disorders vary widely in their presentation, and both *DSM-IV* and *ICD-10* subdivide them into different types. *DSM-IV* divides conduct disorders into childhood onset (onset before 10 years of age), adolescent onset (onset at 10 years of age or older) and oppositional defiant disorder (ODD), characterised by persistently hostile or defiant behaviour outside the normal range, but without aggressive or antisocial behaviour. *ICD-10* divides conduct disorders into socialised conduct disorder, unsocialised conduct disorder, conduct disorders confined to the family context, and ODD.

There are a number of risk factors that can predispose children to conduct disorders. These factors can be environmental, or associated with the family or the child. Environmental risk factors include social disadvantage, homelessness, low socio-economic status, poverty, overcrowding and social isolation (Hausman and Hammen 1993; American Academy of Child and Adolescent Psychiatry 1997; Carr 1999). Family risk factors include marital discord (Marshall and Watt 1999), substance misuse or criminal activities (Frick et al., 1991), and abusive and injurious parenting practices (Luntz and Widom 1994). Children with a 'difficult' temperament, brain damage, epilepsy, chronic illness and cognitive deficits are also more prone to conduct disorders (e.g., Greenberg and Speltz 1993; Prior et al., 1993; Marshall and Watt 1999).

The prevalence of conduct disorders is difficult to estimate because of the judgement involved in distinguishing between them and normal, age-appropriate rebellious/dissocial behaviour. However, it is estimated that in the UK, the prevalence in children aged 5–10 years is 6.9 per cent for boys and 2.8 per cent in girls, of which Oppositional Defiant Disorder (see below) represents 4.5 per cent and 2.4 per cent respectively. In older children (11–16 years of age), the prevalence of diagnosed conduct disorders is slightly higher, at 8.1 per cent for boys and 5.1 per cent for girls, although ODD is less prevalent, at 3.5 per cent and 1.7 per cent respectively (Green et al., 2004).

Although there is a lack of data to produce a full natural history model of conduct disorder – that is, the course that it follows over the life-cycle – there is a substantial amount of evidence to show the negative long-term effects. Thus, the outlook is particularly poor in early onset conduct disorder, reinforcing the importance of early effective treatment. More than 60 per cent of 3 year olds with conduct disorders still exhibit problems at the age of 8 if left untreated, and many problems will persist into adolescence and adulthood (Gould and Richardson 2006). Approximately half of children diagnosed with conduct disorders receive a diagnosis of antisocial personality disorders as adults (American Academy of Child and Adolescent Psychiatry 1997), others being diagnosed with psychiatric disturbances including substance misuse, mania, schizophrenia, obsessive–compulsive disorder, major depressive disorder and panic disorder (Maughan and Rutter 1998).

Conduct disorders have a significant and detrimental impact on the quality of life of both the child and family or carers. Children with conduct disorders are at high risk of experiencing future disadvantage through social exclusion, poor school achievement, long-term unemployment, juvenile delinquency and crime, and poor interpersonal relationships leading to family break-up in adulthood, divorce and abuse of their own children (Rutter and Giller 1983; Robins 1991).

Conduct disorders can be managed through a combination of interventions targeted at both the child and the family. Child-focused therapies include behavioural therapy, cognitive therapy, psychotherapy, social skills training, play therapy, music/art therapy and occupational therapy. Family therapy usually involves a therapist meeting with the whole family to explore personal interactions that may be contributing to or sustaining a child's problem behaviours. However, many children with conduct disorders will not receive treatment because of the limited resources currently available and the high prevalence of the condition, and also the difficulty of engaging some families in treatment (Richardson and Joughin 2002). An appraisal by the National Institute for Health and Clinical Excellence (NICE) of parenting programmes aimed at the management of children under 12 with conduct disorders found that the evidence for the effectiveness of such programmes was strong, provided that they followed various principles, including an approach based on social learning principles (e.g., using role play and 'homework' between sessions), working towards aims that were set by the parents and, not least, providing practical support for parents to attend such programmes, such as crèche facilities (Gould and Richardson 2006). NICE cites as examples of effective programmes, the Webster-Stratton Incredible

Years programme and the 'Triple P' programme, although does not preclude the option of agencies developing their own 'home-grown' programmes provided they follow evidence-based principles and are rigorously evaluated.

In a review of the research relating to effective interventions for conduct disorders in older children, a different picture emerged (Liabo and Richardson 2007). The most promising method of intervention emerging from the evidence-base is family therapy, particularly 'functional family therapy'. One of the most commonly offered interventions for conduct disorders in young people is multisystemic therapy (MST); although the evidence does not suggest it is harmful, MST seems no more effective than 'treatment as usual'. Parenting programmes, effective for younger children, appear to be less successful in modifying the behaviour of adolescents (Liabo and Richardson 2007).

Oppositional defiant disorder

Oppositional defiant disorder (ODD) is a diagnosis most commonly used in relation to younger children and is defined as a milder form of conduct disorder. It is characterised by significantly defiant, disobedient and provocative behaviour, but without the level of aggressive, antisocial behaviour associated with full conduct disorder. Social workers will wish to be alert to the risks of giving young children a psychiatric diagnosis when a child's behaviour is appropriate in terms of normal stages of development. The advice for the management of ODD is as for conduct disorders, with parenting programmes being helpful for parents seeking to cope with a younger child's confrontational behaviour in ways that are constructive and non-punitive.

Attention deficit hyperactivity disorder

Attention deficit hyperactivity disorder (ADHD – also known as hyperkinetic disorder) is a behavioural disorder that is characterised by three core features of inattention, hyperactivity and impulsivity. These problems tend to become apparent in early childhood, and can persist into adulthood. To be considered ADHD as opposed to natural exuberance the problem behaviours need to be 'pervasive' or manifested across contexts – so not only in the home or school, for example – and to be persistent in time, usually for more than six months. The distractibility of children with ADHD and their inability to complete tasks puts them at risk of underachieving at school and consequently of later social disadvantage. Their impulsivity can also lead to personal danger as they are less likely to heed warning signs of risk, and also situations where lack of consideration of negative consequences of behaviour leads them into dissocial behaviour and problems with authority. Children with ADHD may present as fidgety and excitable, though they may not show equal degrees of severity in all three areas of inattention, hyperactivity and impulsivity. NICE's guidelines (National Collaborating Centre for Mental Health 2008) for ADHD advise that a diagnosis of ADHD should not be made unless a moderate degree of psychological, social and/or educational or occupational impairment in multiple settings is demonstrated. The epidemiological research suggests that ADHD is a common problem, and a well-conducted UK survey found a rate of 3.62 per cent amongst boys and 0.85 per cent amongst girls (Ford et al., 2003).

There have been controversies about ADHD as a clinical diagnosis in relation to its validity, with great variation in rates of diagnosis in different countries, particularly the US (National Collaborating Centre for Mental Health 2008: 27), suggesting it is at least partly socially constructed. There has also been concern about the increasing reliance on drugs, particularly the use of psychostimulants such as methylphenidate ('Ritalin'), leading to disquiet that this is a 'chemical cosh' to manage boisterous behaviour. However, evidence-based practice, even within medical psychiatry is seeing a shift towards psychosocial responses to ADHD. NICE's advice recommends that the first line of intervention should be parent–education/training programmes, as for conduct disorders, with psychological support also for the child such as social skills or cognitive behavioural therapy. Only in severe ADHD is medication proposed as a first line treatment, though this is also with assessment of the social and educational context of the problems. As the NICE guideline states:

> Families affected by ADHD will benefit from support from all agencies, such as education, social services, their GP, mental health services and in some cases the youth justice system and police. These agencies can best help families and those with ADHD by working together to offer a package of support for the child/adolescent *and* the family. Medication alone is not the answer; they still require a great deal of support to manage the disorder.
>
> (National Collaborating Centre for Mental Health 2008: 93)

Activity 4.1 Behaviour disorders and social exclusion

Reread the sections on conduct disorders, opposition defiant disorder and attention deficit hyperactivity disorder. Try to identify the forms of social exclusion that a child living with these conditions might experience, and consider what forms of social work intervention might increase their social inclusion.

Developmental disorders

Autism

Autism was first described by Kanner in 1943 as a disorder characterised by three core areas of impairment:

- Impairments in social interaction, particularly problems in making warm relationships with other people, sometimes to the extent that the child appears to make no differentiation between people and objects. The child may appear to resent physical contact, even affectionate touching or hugging by parents, and may seem emotionally indifferent to significant others. This can be very distressing for families. Another feature of autism is avoidance of eye contact, with noticeable levels of gaze avoidance.

- Speech and language disorders, sometimes with complete absence of speech. Sometimes parents report that their child initially appeared to be developing speech normally, but that they then regressed. Where autistic children have speech this often takes the form of 'echolalia', repeating phrases that have just been said to them. Superficially, this can appear like appropriate communication, but is repetition without understanding.

- Obsessive desire for sameness is shown by children with autism both in an inflexible need for constancy in their environment, and by stereotypical repetition of behaviours such as playing with the same toy incessantly, or making gestures repeatedly such as finger flicking in front of the face, from which the child cannot be distracted.

Autism has its onset before the age of three and, as already noted, parents often describe their child as apparently having normal development which then reverses. Early accounts of autism also described this a 'childhood schizophrenia' but this is now regarded as an inappropriate label, as its presentation is distinct from schizophrenia and there is no evidence that autistic children have increased chances of developing schizophrenia in later life. Around 75 per cent of children with autism have learning disabilities (though this can be difficult to assess because of communication problems and short attention spans), and approximately 25 per cent of autistic children develop epilepsy. Media interest and cultural representations (such as the film *The Rainman*) of autistic children as 'savants', individuals who have islands of brilliance such as precocious musical talents or artistic skills, are true only of a very small number of children with autism, and distort popular understanding of the condition. The occurrence of autism is far more common in boys with a ratio of boys to girls of around 4:1. It used to be believed that autism was more prevalent in higher social classes (when the author worked in a specialist unit for autistic children it was part of the 'folklore' amongst staff that the children of middle-class parents were given the diagnosis of autism for their child as being more palatable than – in the 1970s – 'mental handicap') but more recent epidemiological evidence suggests a normal distribution amongst social classes (Burton 2006).

Autism appears to have an organic basis, and early psychological theories that it resulted from problems of attachment to parents, particularly mothers, are now discredited. There has also been misunderstanding arising from research, later also discredited, suggesting that the onset of autism correlated with infants receiving MMR vaccinations (Baron-Cohen 2009). At the present time there is no specific medical treatment for autism. Social workers may play a role within the multidisciplinary team offering family support and education, and helping parents establish behaviour modification approaches to managing their child. Many children with autism will require special education and social workers may also support and advocate for parents in establishing entitlement to services for which their child has an assessed, 'statemented', need.

Asperger's Syndrome

Children with Asperger's Syndrome show some behaviours that overlap with the core features of autism, namely that the quality of their social interaction is impaired, and they have a restricted range of interests and behaviours. However, unlike with autism, they have no significant delay in speech acquisition or cognitive development. As intelligence is not impaired, Asperger's Syndrome tends to be identified later than autism. Because of the similarity to autism, but difference in the degree of impairment, these conditions are sometimes referred to as constituting 'autistic spectrum disorders'. A young person living with Asperger's Syndrome has some caustic comments to make about this:

> Asperger (*sic*) Syndrome comes under the umbrella of autism. That's quite a useful way to think of the autistic spectrum – as an umbrella with lots of people under it all in different places. The trouble with that analogy is that some people are being rained on a lot harder than others and that doesn't really happen with an umbrella.
>
> (Jackson 2002: 20)

The prevalence of the syndrome is difficult to establish, though again there is a preponderance of boys identified, with a ratio to girls of around 6:1. Many of these children and young people will lead successful, independent lives, and their intellectual qualities may assist them in occupations that place a premium on detailed, focused inquiry such as academia. The problems that are associated with Asperger's Syndrome such as difficulty in empathising with the feelings of others, interpreting non-verbal communication, or difficulty in understanding metaphorical language can cause relationship or social difficulties. An understanding by social workers of these challenges can help them to communicate effectively with the person with Asperger's Syndrome.

Emotional disorders

Childhood depression

Until comparatively recently depression was not recognised as something that troubled children; a mainstream psychiatric textbook from 1983 stated:

> However, depressive disorders of the adult type seldom occur before puberty and they are not common even at that age.
>
> (Gelder et al., 1983: 649)

That view has undergone revision. The twelve-month period prevalence estimates for depression are approximately 1 per cent for pre-pubertal children and around 3 per cent for post-pubertal adolescents (Angold and Costello 2001). In pre-pubertal children, there is no sex difference in prevalence, whereas in post-pubertal adolescents the prevalence in females may be higher than that of males, whose prevalence continues to rise but at a much slower rate. The problems can become persistent with 30 per cent of children having further occurrences of depression within five years, and there is evidence that with each recurrence the young person becomes more susceptible to psychosocial factors triggering the next episode (Kendler et al., 2001). Suicide is a real risk, estimated at 3 per cent over the following ten years (Harrington 2001).

Chapter 5

The manifestation of depression in children shows some similarities with adult depression (see Chapter 5), with groups of signs and behaviours around alterations in three core aspects of experience: mood, thinking and activity. Mood changes would include sadness or irritability, loss of pleasure in interests. Thinking may be characterised by inefficiency and high levels of self-criticism, low self-esteem and a feeling that nothing can be done to make circumstances better. Activity is at a relatively low level (though superficially this may be disguised by anxiety or agitation), possibly accompanied by changes in appetite for food (greater or lesser), all of which is reinforced by failure to complete tasks successfully. In severe instances there may be irrational feelings of guilt and desert of punishment, which may be accompanied by thoughts of suicide, which should be taken seriously by a practitioner. Typical scenarios indicating that a young person might be depressed include loss of interest in their appearance, withdrawal, loss of interest in external events and episodes of self-harm.

Surveys of prevalence of depression in children show an association with adverse social factors, indicating scope for social work intervention. In the national survey of child and adolescent mental health (Meltzer et al., 2000), 10 per cent of 5 to 15 year olds had a mental disorder including 4 per cent with emotional disorder (anxiety and depression) and 0.9 per cent with depression. Children and young people with emotional disorders, when compared with those without a mental disorder, were nearly twice as likely to be living with a lone parent (28 per cent versus 15 per cent), more than twice as likely to be with both parents being unemployed (27 per cent versus 12 per cent), and more likely to have parents who were on low incomes, had fewer qualifications and lived in social sector housing (National Collaborating Centre for Mental Health 2005a). Particular circumstances and settings with which childhood depression is particularly associated are:

- school refusal (more often girls who refuse school than boys);

- onset of behavioural difficulties following a disciplinary crisis;

- experience of maltreatment or traumatic experiences such as sexual abuse;

- children and young people who self-harm;

- chronic family disruption;

- persistent drug and alcohol problems.

Research has found that 95 per cent of children and young people with major depression have long-standing psychosocial problems, including family conflict, separation and divorce, domestic violence, physical or sexual abuse, and school-related problems including bullying and social isolation. A smaller number of cases arise from a single, negative event such as an assault (Goodyer et al., 2000).

National practice guidelines stress the importance of psychological and social interventions, rather than a medicalised, drug-based approach (National Collaborating Centre for Mental Health 2005a). They stress the need to assess the social, educational and family environment, including the quality of interpersonal relationships within the family and with peers. NICE's guidance is that social problems should be assessed and managed in collaboration with the wider network of education and social care. If parents have mental health problems, these also need to be addressed. For moderate to severe depression in children and young people, research shows that psychological interventions, including cognitive behavioural therapy, interpersonal therapy or family therapy should be the first line of intervention, delivered by an appropriately trained CAMHS professional, and maintained for at least three months.

Some children are persistently sad, without developing full depression (sometimes described in the medical literature as 'dysphoria') and this is also often associated with longstanding adverse social and environmental factors that may be amenable to social work intervention.

Activity 4.2 Depression and young people

'It is the autumn of 1995: I am 14 years old. Each morning I am meant to get out of bed at 5.45 to catch the school bus, which leaves 50 minutes later. But this hasn't happened in weeks. Instead, I have a new routine. My alarm goes off like a piercing scream; I unplug it and smash my face into my pillow. I am dizzy with fear and can only move in a slow and laboured manner, as if the air in my room has been thickened with gelatin. I listen for the sound of my father's footsteps. He bangs on the door. 'Time to get up,' he says, cautiously. 'Fuck off,' I reply, feeling alarmed that I'm saying this to my father. He sighs and goes to get my mum. Her approach is softer. 'Darling,' she says, standing next to my bed, stroking my hair, 'you really have to get going now. I'll make you some tea.' 'Fuck you,' I say, pushing her away, burrowing deeper under my duvet. I can hear her crying in the hall. I start the first of my own daily floods of tears. I wail for 90 minutes; the bus rolls past. My father pushes and persuades me into his car. Upon arrival, the crying starts again. Dad parks the car and tries to cajole me into going to my lessons. He is gentle, persuasive. Yes, I think, I can do this, I can go to school. But then I put my hand on the door handle and am overwhelmed with the conviction that if I step out of the car I will die. After an hour or so of the back and forth, Dad gives up and takes me home. Or I gather all of my strength and shuffle into my English lesson, telling my friends my face is swollen because of hay fever.'

The above is an article by Jean Hannah Edelstein about her childhood depression (*The Independent*, Tuesday 21 August 2007). What signs of depression are revealed in this extract and how and where would you signpost her and her family for help?

Enuresis

Problems of incontinence sometimes are presented to social workers as they may be contributory factors to family stress and even, in cases where there are severe parenting problems, be a trigger factor in cases of child abuse. For these reasons it is important for social workers to have some understanding of factors involved in incontinence, not least so that where necessary parents can be supported and reassured in their management of the problem. Diagnostic distinctions are conventionally made between nocturnal, diurnal or mixed types depending on the timing of the enuresis, and between primary (if control has never been achieved) and secondary (if enuresis is preceded by a period of control) but many practitioners feel that these distinctions are not of particular help in making an assessment and deciding on an intervention approach. Nevertheless, where the problem does appear to be of a secondary nature it can be helpful to identify whether a stressor has triggered the regression, such as change of school or family upheaval, in which case reassurance around that factor may be more productive than concentrating on the enuresis.

Enuresis can be defined as the involuntary passing of urine in the absence of an organic cause and after the chronological and mental age of 5. Many parents who are anxious about their child's enuresis have unrealistic expectations of their child, and lack understanding of the prevalence of 'accidents' amongst children. At the age of 7, approximately 7 per cent of boys and 3 per cent of girls still have episodes of wetting, particularly at night-time. In most cases it is caused by a delay in the development of the neurological connections necessary for achieving bladder control, hence it is beyond the child's volition to avoid accidents and, indeed, it has a genetic component with late control sometimes being inherited through families.

Social workers will need to have established that there is not an organic (physiological) basis to the problem, such as a urinary tract infection, abnormality of the urinary tract or epilepsy. In the absence of a physical problem in most instances all that is required is an explanation to the parents of the nature of the problem, the need for consistency in their approach, and reassurance that it will resolve. Where the problem is more intractable, a behavioural approach can be introduced such as a star chart to reward dryness or referral for provision of a 'bell and pad' alarm system. The latter operates on the basis of 'classical conditioning' that the pad is placed under the bed sheet and a bell or buzzer is set off when it detects moisture. There is some illogicality to this theoretical explanation as the child does not wake until the 'accident' has begun to occur, and its efficacy is likely to be a product of the therapeutic effects of the additional attention to the child's needs.

Encopresis

Encopresis is more uncommon than enuresis but may cause more distress to the child and family. *DSM-IV* defines it as, 'repeated involuntary passage of faeces into places not appropriate for that purpose . . . the event must take place for at least 3 months, the chronologic age and mental age of the child must be at least 4 years' (American Psychiatric Association 1994). Again, a distinction can be made between primary and secondary forms. If it is primary, that is, bowel control has never been achieved, in most instances this reflects some level of inconsistency in the way that toilet training has been introduced to the child. The family may need support and advice about the introduction of clear routines to the child. Secondary encopresis is more often related to stress arising from the child's environment, or psychological distress leading to defiance. In these instances the main focus of intervention is again likely to be the factor causing stress, along with support to parents to reward the child for re-establishing appropriate toileting.

Elective or selective mutism

Some children who have achieved normal developmental milestones, including speech, may suddenly cease speaking in specific situations, such as school. This is described as selective or elective mutism. Often it is associated with other manifestations of insecurity such as social withdrawal. This behaviour can be immensely frustrating for families or professionals such as teachers, but they can be reassured by the social worker or other members of the team that the situation will resolve itself, although this may take months or even years. Obviously, because mutism is often associated with an environmental trigger such as a change of school, support with resolving the underlying problem should be offered.

Working with parents with mental health problems

Research suggests that in the UK about 4 per cent of all parents have mental health problems and Office of National Statistics psychiatric morbidity data shows the pervasiveness of mental distress across all social groups and types of household, including those with and without children (Gould 2006c). However, the excess of mental distress amongst lone parents is noteworthy and has been the subject of further studies (Targosz et al., 2003). These show that there is a higher rate of mental disorder of all types among lone parents than for adults living as a couple with children. Lone parents are almost three times more likely than couples with children to have more serious functional psychoses (this includes disorders such as schizophrenia and bipolar affective disorder) or drug dependence, and are nearly twice as likely as couples with children to have a neurotic disorder. In their secondary analysis of data from the British National Survey of Psychiatric Morbidity, to look at lone parenthood, depression and social exclusion, Targosz et al. (2003) confirmed that lone mothers had prevalence rates of depressive episodes of 7 per cent, roughly three times higher than any other group. These increased rates of depressive conditions were not apparent after controlling for measures of social disadvantage, stress and isolation. The authors concluded that the high rates of material disadvantage and of depressive disorder had considerable implications for mental health and social policy. This data from community-based surveys confirms the messages from Brown and Harris's (1978) classic study of working-class women in Camberwell, that the coincidence of social stressors such as lack of a supportive relationship, poor housing conditions and caring for young children at home can create susceptibility to depression, triggered by adverse life events. Social workers need to be alert to these vulnerabilities and see the importance of supporting parents to access social support and alleviate material stress in order to protect against common mental health problems such as depression. It is troubling that Sheppard's research found that social workers had a lack of awareness of the effects of depression on confidence and self-esteem, which undermined the relationships that social workers were trying to establish with mothers (Sheppard 2001). The same study showed that depressed mothers valued social workers persisting with contact even when the former struggled – because of the depression – to respond.

The extent to which the mental health of a parent impacts on their children will depend on a number of factors, including the duration and severity of the mental health problems (a short period of depression will have less impact on family life than a chronic, psychotic disorder), whether there is a well parent to manage the periods of difficulty experienced by the unwell parent, and the child's own resilience and personality. A summary of the research in this area for the National Society for the Prevention of Cruelty To Children (Green 2002) is provided in Box 4.2.

Box 4.2 A summary of the effects of parental mental health problems for parenting and child welfare (based on Green 2002)

- *Effects on parenting.* Often parents who experience mental health problems feel that this has an adverse affect on the quality of their parenting. Ethier et al. (1995), for instance, found that clinically depressed mothers were more likely to speak less often to children, enforce obedience unilaterally and react in more hostile and irritable fashion. Murray (1996) produced similar findings of social disadvantage, relationship problems with children and the latter having increased levels of behaviour difficulties. There is some risk of pathologising mothers who are depressed (White 1996) and it is not clear that all these studies are methodologically rigorous.

- *Direct effects on children.* There is some controversy over whether the presence of parental mental health problems elevates the level of risk to a child of abuse. Early commentators on child abuse such as Kempe saw abuse as inherently a psychiatric, medicalised problem. More recently there has been a move away from this medicalisation of abuse, seeing it as complex and multifactorial. Reviews of deaths of children at the hands of their parents have found over-representation of parents with mental health problems (Falkov 1995) but these are not representative samples. As Rutter (1989) has commented, the more frequent risk to children comes from psychological adversity as a result to interruptions to the formations of attachments, development and mental health.

- *Children's role as carers.* Some children find themselves in the role of care for a parent with a mental health problem, the numbers are difficult to estimate but Dearden and Becker (1995) estimated that there could be between 10,000 and 40,000 children in a caring role, and approximately one-third of these were looking after a parent with a mental health problem. Aldridge and Beckers' (2003) subsequent qualitative research has given voice to young people about their experiences of caring for a parent with a mental health problem. The term 'young carer' is itself problematic as the young person may or may not be willing to perform the role, or the 'young carer' label may disguise the situation where the caring is imposed by the lack of provision of services for the parent. Among the risks to the young person is the denial of the educational and social experiences necessary for their appropriate development.

In addition to Green's typology can be added the effects of parental mental health on child poverty; as well as complicating everyday parenting tasks, mental health problems in parents contribute to family poverty. Mental illness is an under-recognised but significant contributory factor to child poverty (Tunnard 2004). There is a lack of hard data but it is likely that there are approximately 1.25 million children in England and Wales living with parents or carers who have a mental health problem (Gould 2006c). Given the huge over-representation of people with mental health problems among those who are out of work, as discussed in Chapter 2 (only 24 per cent of people with long-term mental health problems are in employment), and amongst recipients of sickness and disability benefits (larger than the total number of recipients of Jobseekers' Allowance in England), it is a reasonable presumption that this situation must be producing hardship for many children. The conservative estimate made by the author in research undertaken for the Joseph Rowntree Foundation was that in 2005 more than 368,000 children lived in poor families where the mental health problems of parents were a contributory factor to their poverty (Gould 2006c).

Chapter 2

Bridging mental health services for children and adults

Many of the mental health difficulties for young people described in this chapter do not magically go away when the young person reaches the age of 17 or 18; for instance behavioural disorders such as conduct disorder or ADHD continue to impair the lives as adults and may be associated with the emergence of forms of mental disorder that characteristically have their onset in early adulthood, such as schizophrenia (Richardson and Joughlin 2002; Liabo and Richardson 2007). There is longstanding frustration on the part of individuals and families that the separation of health and social care services into adult and children's services creates a transition point at which the individual is either lost to view or becomes subject to boundary disputes as to whose responsibility they are. This issue has been recognised at a policy level but securing action to safeguard young people from falling through the safety net is elusive. A Department of Health (2006b) report, *Transitions*, acknowledged the problem but explicitly excluded mental health services from its remit:

> While there are similar concerns about how best to improve the transitions between CAMHS and adult mental health services, there are a number of current developments in CAMHS provision, notably improving the access to services for 16 and 17 year olds and the development of services providing early intervention for young people with psychoses which requires a partnership between CAMHS and adult mental health services
>
> (Department of Health 2006b: 6)

The apparent complacency of this report is undermined by the report's own evidence, citing examples of areas where CAMHS terminated responsibility for children at 16 and adult mental services would not accept referrals for individuals below the age of 18 (Department of Health 2006b: 40). Unsurprisingly, a more recent review of CAMHS has commented:

> smooth transitions to young adulthood are still not being achieved and there is considerable variation around the country. This includes transitions to a range of services, including adult mental health services, housing, support services in colleges and universities and adult social care.
>
> (CAMHS Review 2008: para. 6.5)

The challenge of bridging the gap between children and adult services should not only fall to CAMHS, it is clear that mental well-being is part of the agenda of a broad range of social initiatives, and social workers are part of or relate to many of those cited in the introduction to this chapter, including Sure Start, Children's Centres, Extended Schools and programmes to improve behaviour and the social and emotional aspects of learning within schools (SEAL). The evidence-base for successful models of transition working is inconclusive (Department of Health 2006b: 25) but there are some generic principles that are applicable to this situation: avoidance of discrimination against young people, which is the outcome where the focus is on avoiding responsibility for an individual rather than looking at their holistic needs; attention to the importance of families as most young people receiving services will still be living with parents or carers, and the mutual rights and needs of both have to be considered; and, teamwork so that professionals work together to follow through the needs of young people as they move into adulthood.

Key points

- Mental health problems are more prevalent in children than has often been recognised by professionals. Many of these problems, if not ameliorated, lead to adverse social outcomes and continuing difficulties in adulthood.

- The National Service Framework for Children, Young People and Maternity Services establishes evidence-based standards for services for children and young people with mental health problems.

- The main reason for referral of children to CAMHS is conduct disorders; research suggests that for younger children with conduct disorders the most effective intervention is parent education and training programmes, though these are less effective as children get older.

- There is a role for social workers in relation to children with developmental disorders by supporting families and advocating with and for them to access appropriate services.

- Emotional disorders in children often respond to psychosocial interventions and these often are valid and evidence-based alternatives to pharmacological treatments.

- The mental health needs of parents should not be overlooked, not least because parents' mental health problems are a factor in child poverty.

Key reading

Gould, N. and Richardson, J. (2006) 'Parent training/education programmes in the management of children with conduct disorders: developing an integrated evidence base for health and social care', *Journal of Children's Services*, 1(4): 47–60.

Meltzer, H., Gatward, R. with Goodman, R. and Ford, T. (2000) The *Mental Health of Children and Adolescents in Great Britain. The report of a survey carried out in 1999 by Social Survey Division of the Office for National Statistics on behalf of the Department of Health, the Scottish Health Executive and the National Assemby for Wales*, London: The Stationery Office.

Tunnard, R. (2004) *Parental Mental Health Problems: key messages from research, policy and practice*, Dartington: Research In Practice.

5 Mental health social work with adults: mood disorders and post-traumatic stress disorder

By the end of this chapter you should have an understanding of:

- An overall appreciation of the nature of mood disorders in adults

- Depression, including its presentation, social factors with which it is associated, and evidence-based approaches to treatment

- Practice implications of working with women experiencing post-natal depression

- Bipolar disorder, including its presentation, social consequences, treatment and the role for social work intervention

- Phobic anxiety and panic disorders, including different forms of phobia, their impact on social functioning and the role of psychosocial interventions

- Post-traumatic stress disorder, social groups at risk of developing the disorder, implications for working with victims of abuse, and interventions to support those affected.

Depression

Depression is one of the most commonly used terms to describe someone's mental state, 'I'm really depressed today' or 'He's suffering from depression'. Clearly, it has connotations for the lay person of indicating low mood but is used without very much precision; little differentiation is made between a transient feeling of unhappiness and a serious and persistent problem that leads to a person seeking help. *ICD-10* groups together a range of conditions described as depressive episode, recurrent depressive episode and mixed anxiety and depressive disorder, and *DSM-IV* uses a similar system of classification. What links these disorders under the umbrella of depression is a range of mental health problems characterised by low mood and loss of enjoyment or interest in everyday events, and an associated range of emotional, cognitive, physical and behavioural signs (National Collaborating Centre for Mental Health 2004: 14). Making a clear differentiation between the lay understanding of depression and a state of mind that reaches a clinical threshold of diagnosis as a clinical condition is elusive; the boundary is permeable but depends on judgement about the severity and intractability of the person's mood. *ICD-10* categorises depression according to the number of symptoms that an individual presents as to whether it is mild, moderate, severe or psychotic. This appears a very reductionist approach based on seemingly arbitrary judgements about thresholds. In its guidance for the management of depression in primary and secondary settings NICE suggests that the categories of recurrent, treatment resistant, chronic, atypical and psychotic depression could be more useful (National Collaborating Centre for Mental Health 2004: 49).

Typically, a person who is depressed has a persistent absence of positive affect in response to events, and this negative affect will recur daily, often with a pattern of low mood in the morning which improves to a degree as the day goes on, though returning by next morning. The person may temporarily have their mood lifted when something agreeable happens, but this lightening of mood is soon replaced by a return to low spirits. Behavioural and physical signs of depression include: an interrupted sleep pattern (often with early waking), irritability, social withdrawal, loss of appetites including food and sex, chronic feelings of fatigue, lower levels of activity, and increased experience of pain, including pains brought on by muscular tension.

Other aspects of thinking on the part of the person with depression are feelings of low self-esteem, guilt and self-blame, sometimes accompanied by thoughts that the person deserves punishment, loss of confidence and inability to influence external events. Unsurprisingly, all this may be accompanied by thoughts of suicide ('suicidality' or 'suicidal ideation'). It has been estimated that two-thirds of suicides occur in people who have depression (Sartorius 2001). Cognitive changes (which as we shall see have become a focus for developing therapeutic interventions) include a preponderance of negative and self-defeating thoughts, low levels of concentration, slowing of mental processes and rumination about negative events in one's life (Cassano and Fava 2002). All this is complicated by the fact that some people with depression feel large amounts of anxiety and their agitated behaviour may not always conform to the classical picture of depression as a state of lethargy and inactivity. This may be particularly significant for the social worker assessing an older person; the presentation of depression does vary with age and the older person's agitation may mask an underlying state of depression. Whether someone has a primary diagnosis of depression or anxiety disorder is a matter of judgement rather than any categorical, clear-cut distinction.

In relatively rare instances of severe depression, a person may have abnormal mental experiences involving hallucinations or delusions, and these may or may not exhibit content that is suggestive of depressive thoughts such as self-blame. In these circumstances it may be difficult for a psychiatrist to make a differential diagnosis between schizophrenia and depression.

The social context of depression is important, and part of the social work role in multidisciplinary settings will be to assess social factors that are relevant, and to intervene to ameliorate them where this is possible. Family relations can be placed under strain when a member is depressed, and a depressed parent may find that their capacity for caring for children is impaired (Ramchandani and Stein 2003). The NICE guideline on the management of depression provides a useful synthesis of socio-demographic factors associated with the condition (National Collaborating Centre for Mental Health 2004). Gender and ethnicity are important variables, though their effects are further complicated by variations over the life course. Depression affects women more than men until around the age of 55, after which men have higher rates of depression. Marriage or cohabitation seems to offer some protection with the highest rates amongst people who are separated, next highest amongst widowed males and divorced females, and lowest prevalence amongst people who are married. Caring for children is associated with higher rates of depression, with lone parents having the highest rates, followed by married parents and individuals who are part of a couple without children having the lowest rates. However, there are some controversies about these estimations as the higher rates for groups such as lone parents may disappear when controlled for socio-economic factors such as income and unemployment. Differences between men and women in their help-seeking behaviour may also be a factor in explaining differential rates of diagnosis.

Men from black and minority ethnic groups do not seem to have higher rates of depression than other males, but significantly higher rates of depression are found for some women, particularly from Asian and Oriental backgrounds. Some caution is necessary in interpreting these findings as they tend to be based on surveys with small samples (Meltzer et al., 1995).

Other social conditions that have risks of higher incidence of depression, drawing on data from the ONS survey of psychiatric conditions (Meltzer et al., 1995), include:

- Unemployment, particularly for women, carries higher risks of depression, with full-time employment being a significant protective factor.

- Membership of lower social classes (3 or below) is associated with higher rates of depression.

- Housing tenure correlates with rates of depression, with those in rented accommodation having higher levels.

- Additional years spent in education reduce the risks of depression, particularly for men.

- Higher levels of depression are found in urban areas than rural.

- Rates of depression are particularly high amongst people who are homeless, with rates estimated for those accommodated in hostels and leased accommodation as around 25 per cent, and as high as 60 per cent amongst the roofless.

- Asylum seekers are a further group with multiple risk factors relating to depression.

As with all statistics drawn from cross-sectional surveys, that is, with data collected at one point in time, we cannot ascribe causality to the relationship between the social circumstances identified above and depression. In particular, practitioners must beware of the 'ecological fallacy', that is, taking evidence about social groups and communities and applying it mechanistically to individuals. Some unemployed, lone parents living in rented accommodation will not be depressed, but knowledge of the research base in relation to at-risk groups will sensitise the practitioner to factors that may be significant in the individual case. Furthermore, there is additional evidence and theoretical reasons for seeing social circumstances as causative in depression. Brown and Harris' (1978) research into causes of depression in working-class women showed that social stress factors created vulnerability to depression, which was then often triggered by a negative life event.

Treatments and their social implications

It should be borne in mind by social workers that most people who experience depression will have recovered within six months, and half of them will not have a recurrence. However, this should not detract from the risks that are present while a person is depressed, nor that there is considerable variation in the course of depression between individuals. For the 50 per cent who do have a recurrence there is an increasing probability of depression returning, 70 per cent at second occurrence and 90 per cent at third recurrence (Kupfer 1991). People who experience depression in early life have higher recurrence of mental health problems (Giles et al., 1989), and outcomes are also poor for older people who develop depression (Cole et al., 1999). Recurrences of episodes of depression may follow a pattern; it is now established that some people are susceptible to seasonal patterns of low mood (seasonal affective disorder), for others there may be patterns related to earlier life events that emerge from compiling a careful social assessment such as anniversaries of significant events such as bereavement.

Community surveys suggest that most people who are depressed do not seek professional help, and when they do general practitioners are very variable in their skills of detecting depression and often it is undetected by them (Goldberg and Huxley 1992). This volume is primarily concerned with social aspects of mental health, but it is useful for social workers to understand some of the social implications of physical treatments. Conversely, the selection of treatment methods by doctors should also take into account social factors, possibly identified in multidisciplinary teams by the social worker:

> When assessing a person with depression, healthcare professionals should consider the psychological, social, cultural and physical characteristics of the patient and the quality of interpersonal relationships. They should consider the impact of these on the depression and the implications for choice of treatment and its subsequent monitoring.
>
> (National Collaboration Centre for Mental Health 2004: 25)

For over forty years the front line of pharmacological intervention for depression has been antidepressants, with several generations of drugs being developed. Tricyclic anti-depressants appeared in the 1950s but were problematic because of their potential to produce allergic reactions and high level of mortality when patients overdosed, a particular danger given the elevated risks of suicide with depression. The more recent family of drugs, the specific serotonin reuptake inhibitors (SSRIs) such as fluoxetine, appeared to offer more efficacious treatment with fewer risks for patients but there are continuing controversies surrounding the efficacy of all these drugs. When allowance is made for the very high placebo effect that occurs when taking any drug for a psychiatric condition, some commentators have questioned whether there is a statistically significant level of improvement from taking anti-depressants (Kirsch 2000). There are also questions about the completeness of the published evidence-base; most drug trials are funded by their manufacturers and it is not always clear whether studies that have negative outcomes (including suicides or other extreme behaviours) have been published (Lexchin et al., 2003).

Although many people experiencing depression will continue to report benefit from taking antidepressants, and some doctors will find this the most convenient way to respond to their patients' requests for help, evidence-based approaches to the management of depression now pay increased attention to non-pharmacological interventions, as indicated by the NICE guidelines cited above. This involves 'stepped care' from initial 'watchful waiting' to see whether the person spontaneously feels better over the course of a few weeks (though excluding those who present as severely depressed who may be psychotic or suicidal), through brief psychological interventions, physical exercise and guided self-help for mild depression, through social support, psychological interventions and drug treatment for moderate depression, and complex psychological intervention, anti-depressant drugs and other physical treatments for severe depression.

Treatment for severe depression may involve Electro Convulsive Treatment (ECT) about which many social workers still feel very uneasy, including those who are involved in compulsory admissions to hospital who consider they may be consigning a service user to this form of treatment. This also continues to be the concern of some service user groups (Rose et al., 2003). Advocates for ECT argue that it is now a very different procedure from that usually depicted in the anti-psychiatry literature which reflected practices where general anaesthetics and muscle relaxants were not used, leading to physical injury and cognitive impairment. Current practice involves both general anaesthetic and muscle relaxants so that the person is not conscious during the procedure and does not experience the convulsions that previously produced injuries such as biting of the tongue. Placing electrodes on one side of the head (the non-dominant side of the brain) also reduces impairment to memory and other cognitive functions.

A review of the effectiveness of ECT (National Institute for Clinical Excellence 2003) produced complex findings; it confirmed that ECT did produce cognitive impairment though this was related to the 'dose' (number of sessions), but that this was not normally permanent, and that ECT was more effective in alleviating depression than some drugs. The overall recommendation of the review was that ECT should be restricted to achieving rapid improvement of severe depression when other methods had been tried. The guidance is that informed consent to ECT should be obtained where possible. Social workers may take it on themselves to ensure that individual's wishes and rights are properly upheld in this respect through advance directives, consultation with carers, advocacy services and the legal protections of the Mental Health Act.

Cognitive behavioural therapies

There are many explanatory theories for the occurrence of depression, ranging from those that are biologically deterministic, stressing genetic heritance, through the models that indicate a relationship between genetic vulnerability and stress factors, through to those which are located in social and psychological models of explanation. Psychodynamic theories emphasise the primacy of early relation-ships and their subsequent influence on emotional resilience, particularly the impact of disruptions to early attachment.

Later approaches have followed the cognitive revolution in psychology, particularly the emergence of cognitive behavioural therapies (CBT); the generic feature of cognitive therapies is the assertion that psychological disturbance arises from the faulty information processing habits that individuals have learned – regardless of the stage of their development at which they were learned – and the idea that these can be unlearned, replacing them with more flexible, helpful ways of thinking. The key figure in the development of CBT for depression was Aaron Beck. Beck noted that people who became depressed had core beliefs or automatic ways of thinking that were typically negative and self-defeating (Beck et al., 1979). These modes of thinking also 'set people up to fail' as they created expectations in life that could never be achieved.

The 'Mental Health First Aid' programme (CSIP/NIMHE, undated) cites the following as examples of depressive thinking:

- I'm a failure

- I have let everyone down

- It's all my fault

- Nothing good ever happens to me

- I'm worthless

- No-one loves me

- I am so alone

- Life is not worth living

- There is nothing good out there

- Things will always be bad.

Later Beck suggested that these modes of habitual thinking could be categorised into two personality styles (Beck 1983). Some depressive people were 'sociotropic', that is, they had unusually high levels of need for approval and acceptance from others, and in order to achieve this approval would constantly prioritise securing that approval in front of meeting their own needs. When these sociotropic tendencies are pursued excessively the resulting denial to oneself of satisfaction of needs becomes depressive in its effect. The second depressive personality style is 'autonomous'; these are people who place unreasonable expectations on their own capacity to achieve goals alone without the help of others. Both styles make the individual highly exposed to disappointment and depression, either because relationships are disrupted or threatened (the sociotropic type) or successful achievement of goals does not materialise, perhaps through educational or career disappointments (the autonomous type).

Mulhern et al. (2004) have helpfully described the steps involved in their approach to CBT when working with people of both types who are depressed:

- *Initial contact and making a therapeutic alliance.* At the point at which the person with depression seeks help they may have been in distress for some time, and the act of seeking help may compound feelings of failure and low self-esteem. They may have adapted their lifestyle to avoid situations that engender depression, perhaps withdrawing from work or social interaction. Mulhern et al. stress the importance of maintaining a non-judgemental response in establishing a therapeutic rapport, and being ready to listen to the person's experience of their depression rather than compiling 'checklists' of symptoms.

- *Assessment.* Again, empathetic engagement is at the heart of the assessment process, and through listening to the narratives that the person gives of their situation, the practitioner draws out the circumstances that seem to be sustaining the episodes of depression, the factors that precipitate depressive feelings and how they normally cope with them. This is also likely to elicit the cognitive strategies the person employs to cope that induce depression, for instance attributing their redundancy to personal inadequacy rather than external economic forces. Assessment will include asking the person to monitor their own activities over a period of time, such as a week, as this then produces a realistic baseline measurement against which improvement and change can be monitored.

- *Behavioural interventions – task assignment.* From this assessment the practitioner and service user can begin to identify a gradual schedule of tasks or activities that they can attempt that will build confidence and moderate their feelings of depression. CBT, like other interventions based on social learning theory, emphasise the importance of 'homework', assignments that the person undertakes in between therapeutic sessions, through which new modes of thinking are tested out, and learning is generalised beyond the therapeutic session to the 'real world'. Assignments are agreed with the person so that they are relevant to their own perception of their problems, and not imposed by the therapist. They are also vehicles for examining core beliefs that have engendered depression, and developing new ways of thinking that are realistic and not self-defeating.

- *Monitoring intervention.* Monitoring and assessment are integral to any behavioural or cognitive behavioural intervention, treating the intervention as an experiment based on a hypothesis of what needs to change and measuring the results. This may take the form of repeating the exercise of keeping a diary of activities. Alternatively, it may involve utilising a validated scale such as Beck's own depression inventory (Beck 1996), though use of such instruments remains rare in the repertoire of social workers, compared to clinical psychologists.

There is perhaps a danger in seeing CBT as a panacea. At present it is in the ascendancy, supported by the UK government's interest in CBT as an intervention for common mental health problems, notably though the Improving Access To Psychological Therapies Programme (Department of Health 2008b). There are also reviews of the evidence advocating the use of CBT across the full range of levels of depression. National clinical guidelines for the management of depression suggest a more nuanced approach proposing that for moderate, severe and treatment-resistant depression CBT should be the psychological approach of choice. However, for mild to moderate depression CBT might be one of a variety of short-term approaches that can be effective, such as problem-solving therapy and counselling (National Collaborating Centre for Mental Health 2004).

Other social work interventions

It can be argued that psychological therapies, though these can be delivered by appropriately trained and supervised social workers, tend to individualise the nature of depression and marginalise the more structural causes of depression. Feeling depressed may be a rational response to external forms of oppression such as racism, poverty or domestic violence. As we have seen, depression is associated with structural forms of disadvantage, although there are individuals within oppressed social groups whose own resilience factors, including their cognitive style, protect them from becoming depressed.

People who have long-term chronic depression may well have problems of sustaining paid employment. This is as work provides structure, social contact and benefits to self-esteem, all of which are important aspects of recovery. Social workers may be able to connect people with chronic depression to befriending schemes, which have been found to be beneficial as part of rehabilitation. Also, liaison with specialist employment services can be effective in supporting people through the transition of finding and returning to work.

Although social support is frequently referred to as a good thing in relation to depression, and social isolation is associated with poor outcomes and chronicity, there has been little attempt to specify what this means, and to evaluate the effectiveness of interventions to reduce isolation. The use of the voluntary sector or informal support structures would, a priori, seem to be of benefit and encouraging people to engage with self-help and voluntary groups also seems intrinsically to be useful. The higher prevalence of depression in women from some black and ethnic minority groups, notably Asian and Oriental (Meltzer et al., 1995), also underlines the importance of supporting statutory and voluntary initiatives directed towards meeting their needs.

Activity 5.1 Depression and parenting

Eileen is a lone parent living in a housing association flat with two children aged 4 and 2. She used to have a well-paid job in a travel agency but left this because of the problems of finding affordable care for her children. Her extended family lives over 50 miles away and she does not have her own transport. Lately, Eileen has found it increasingly difficult to motivate herself to care adequately for the children, with mealtimes becoming erratic and little overall daily routine. She is irritable with the children and small frustrations make her tearful.

All this is told to you when she calls into a family resource centre to inquire about local child care resources. What are the factors that research suggests may be contributing to Eileen's low mood? What kinds of intervention might a social worker make to alleviate her mental state?

Post-natal depression – social work implications

An additional type of depression which has relevance for social workers, particularly those operating in services for children and families, is post-natal depression. It is estimated that depression occurs in about 10 to 15 per cent of mothers in the month after giving birth (Demott et al., 2006), though its recognition may be complicated by the presentation of tiredness, irritability and anxiety rather than classic signs of depression. Post-natal depression has potential consequences not only for the mother but also the subsequent development of her children: the children of women who experience depression have an increased likelihood of subsequent referral to Child and Adolescent Mental Health Services and suffer mental health problems in later life (Demott et al., 2006). The same review of the evidence in relation to post-natal depression found that social isolation of pregnant women is a risk factor and that intervention to provide support might have a preventative effect, though the evidence is inconclusive.

Many more women experience 'post-natal blues', a milder form of unhappiness in the first few days after giving birth. This tends to resolve itself and current evidence-based guidance is that professional intervention is not typically needed, although reassurance may be given that the feelings are transient

(Demott et al., 2006). This contrasts with the other end of the spectrum: a small proportion of women who experience post-natal disturbance that is so severe that it is a form of psychosis, 'puerperal psychosis'. The condition is precipitated by puerperal sepsis (infection of the genital tract after childbirth). Though this is now rare given the effectiveness of antibiotics, the condition is often of sufficient severity that an approved professional such as a social worker may need to apply for the mother to be compulsorily admitted to hospital, ideally to a unit where continuity of contact with the baby can be maintained. Puerperal psychosis may take the form of bipolar affective disorder (see below), delirium, or it may present as schizophrenia ('schizophreniform'). Given that the newborn baby may become incorporated in the delusional thinking of the mother, social workers need to consider potential risk to the child. There are high probabilities of puerperal psychosis recurring following subsequent births, so where women have a history of this condition, then proactive steps may be taken to monitor and support them and thereby protect their children.

Bipolar disorder

Sometimes depression may be referred to as 'unipolar affective disorder', meaning a disturbance of mood that is experienced at one end of the continuum of emotionality that runs from very low to very elated feelings. The other end of the spectrum is described as mania. People who experience alternating high and low moods have in the past been described as experiencing 'manic-depression', although the preferred contemporary term is 'bipolar disorder', sometimes also referred to as 'bipolar affective disorder'. Bipolar disorder is a cyclical mood disorder that involves periods of serious interruptions to mood and behaviour, interspersed with periods of relatively stable and unimpaired functioning. The defining feature of bipolar disorder is periods of hypomania or mania, that is, expansive and grandiose affect and driven behaviour which if unmodified leads to exhaustion. The individual may also have periods of major depression, though the diagnosis of bipolar disorder, in both *ICD-10* and *DSM-IV*, requires that the person has experienced an episode of mania, and cannot be made solely on the basis of depressive episodes.

Sometimes mental distress is romanticised by the popular media, in the sense that individuals may be depicted as having heightened levels of sensitivity, or insight into a 'mad' world. In that mania and bipolar affective disorder seem to be disproportionately diagnosed amongst artists and other creative people, this sometimes diminishes or distracts from the anguish and despair that it can cause in people's lives. For every celebrity such as the late Spike Milligan and Stephen Fry who seem able to harness their mood fluctuations to perform and entertain, there are many more individuals whose lives can be catastrophically disrupted.

In the early stages of mania a person can seem the life and soul of the party, highly engaging and gregarious, able to make quick word plays and impulsively generous. This can then give way to highly inappropriate behaviour where judgement about social norms is seriously impaired. The person can be grandiose, overbearing and highly irritable, if not aggressive, when their behaviour is challenged. Mania is often accompanied by 'pressure of speech', speaking without pause as if the person has lost the capability to turn off their outpouring of words. The content of such speech may reveal delusions of grandeur, imagining they have influence and authority considerably beyond their actual social position. Most damaging of all for the individual's self-esteem and respect, their behaviour can become highly impulsive and disinhibited. This may lead to sexual relationships that the person would never countenance in their everyday lives, acts of reckless disinhibition such as taking off clothes in public and extravagant impulses such as spending sprees leading to debt and insolvency. The by-products of these forms of behaviour can be loss of employment, breakdown of family and other close relationships and long-term social consequences, such as homelessness.

The mean average age for the onset of mania and bipolar affective disorder is 21, although this should not be interpreted rigidly as there is considerable variation (Lloyd et al., 2005). Most prevalence studies have found even distribution of the condition between sexes. Studies have found a higher incidence of bipolar disorder amongst black and minority ethnic groups, and higher rates of hospitalisation, as for schizophrenia (Kennedy et al., 2004; Lloyd et al., 2005). Caution needs to be exercised in interpreting these findings about ethnicity; they may reflect increased difficulties that people from minorities have in accessing services until their condition has deteriorated, along with simultaneously coping with the social pressures of social exclusion and racism.

Of all the major forms of mental disorder, bipolar disorder seems to be the most heritable, with a 79 per cent concordance rate between identical twins, compared to 19 per cent in non-identical twins (Craddock and Jones 1999; McGuffin et al., 2003). These rates hold up for twins who are raised separately. Despite the evidence for this strong biological basis for mania and bipolar affective disorder, there does also seem to be a causal role played by psychosocial events in the initial onset of the disorder. Many individuals experience their first episode in the context of severe stress or following major negative life events, and the pattern of recurrence of episodes may follow a seasonal pattern, perhaps determined by anniversaries of these precipitating events.

Despite the florid and sometimes bizarre nature of an individual's presentation with mania, the serious hazards of the condition should not be underestimated: when experiencing a manic episode, individuals can severely neglect their own welfare, leading to dehydration and malnourishment; dressing inappropriately or unseasonably for harsh weather conditions can result in hypothermia; and lack of sleep for prolonged periods can lead to severe exhaustion and even death. For these reasons, coupled with the difficulties of engaging with a person who is very manic in order to persuade them of other courses of action, an admission to hospital for initial treatment may be unavoidable. Social workers acting as applicants for compulsory admission to hospital will need to take into account the potentially serious outcomes of untreated episodes of mania.

The main pharmacological maintenance treatment for bipolar affective disorder and acute manic episodes is lithium, even though the mechanism by which the drug works is poorly understood (National Collaboration Centre for Mental Health 2006b). Lithium also has a range of side effects including weight gain, gastrointestinal disturbance and skin disorders. Not least, if the dosage is not titrated, that is, introduced gradually until a therapeutic dosage is reached, irreversible kidney damage can be caused, and six monthly testing of kidney function is required. Although lithium is effective in stabilising mood and preventing manic or depressive episodes for many who take it, the reasons are also clear why some people prefer not to accept medication and to take their chances with their mood disorder. In the United States the most commonly used mood stabiliser is valproate, which is quicker acting than lithium, and thought to be more effective for stabilising people with rapidly fluctuating bipolar affective disorder, but again there are unpleasant side effects such as nausea, weight gain and tremor. Valproate is potentially dangerous when prescribed for women of childbearing age as it can cause foetal malformation (National Collaborating Centre for Mental Health 2006b).

Although the main emphasis in the management of bipolar affective disorder and recurrent mania is on drug treatments, the role of psychosocial intervention should not be overlooked. If an individual has children but is without support networks when they become disturbed, there may be a need to help make arrangement for the care of children. An episode of mania may last for several months, but typically individuals regain their personality and faculties unimpaired once the abnormal mood subsides. They may then need supportive counselling to deal with their feelings of shame and regret if their behaviour has been inappropriate of hurtful to others. Their financial affairs may have been affected, with debt accrued through shopping sprees, and practical advice about sorting out their affairs may be welcomed, perhaps with referral to an agency such as the Citizen's Advice Bureau. In addition to all this there is a role for education for the individual and family members about the nature of the condition and its possible consequences. Not least, individuals and families may be encouraged to learn to avoid triggers such as over-work, sleep deprivation and substance misuse, and to recognise the early signs of mood instability, with the hope that at that point the person has sufficient insight to seek help. Introduction to support or self-help groups may also be of help.

Anxiety and phobias

Like depression, anxiety is a mental state with which most people can identify, to some degree. Most people, in anticipation of a challenging situation such as taking an examination or giving a public performance, feel some level of psychological and physiological disturbance which they might label as 'anxiety'. For many the experience of anxiety, provided it is under their control and within the limits of what they can tolerate, is seen as something that is positive as it improves their performance or 'raises their game'. In evolutionary terms anxiety plays a role in triggering fight or flight responses that take an individual out of threatening situations, or reinforces their resolve to face down threats successfully. Anxiety, then, is apprehension in the face of a perceived threat, although that threat may be external and situational (e.g., brought about by confined spaces or exposure to a feared object such as a spider) or internal (e.g., generalised anxiety states, panic disorder or obsessive compulsive disorder).

Anxiety is problematic when it is experienced as overwhelming, and the avoidance of situations that provoke anxiety starts to severely compromise the range of activities such as work or leisure that the person undertakes. Anxiety that is disabling may involve experiencing a combination of unpleasant experiences that are physiological (trembling, perspiring, dryness of mouth, muscle tension, sickness, gastric disturbance, rapid pulse), behavioural (running away or avoiding a situation) and psychological (feelings of fear, dread and apprehension). Once again, most people recognise some degree of these reactions to everyday stressful events, but for the person whose lives are blighted by anxiety, the intensity of these signs of anxiety can be completely overwhelming, to the extent that they genuinely feel they are about to die. In psychiatry, anxiety states are commonly referred to as neuroses, although the latter has come to have very pejorative connotations in common discourse, and to describe someone as 'neurotic' is often a way of dismissing an individual's problems, often without understanding the depth of their distress.

Sometimes someone may be simultaneously both depressed and anxious, and the management of their problems will depend on which seems to be the most dominant of their mental states. Some people may have a 'generalised anxiety state', free-floating anxiety where they have elevated feelings of anxiety most of the time, without any identifiable trigger. Many people with generalised anxiety problems will not come to the attention of helping agencies but when they do then counselling, or cognitive behavioural therapy, might be helpful. A medical practitioner might prescribe a drug such as benzodiazepine but unless this is short term there can be problems of dependency.

Phobic anxiety and panic disorders

Sometimes an individual may develop a persistent and irrational fear in relation to an object, activity or situation such that they experience high levels of anticipatory anxiety which results in them avoiding that which is feared. Where this overwhelming fear and avoidance behaviours become so entrenched that they impair someone's quality of life, this can be referred to as a phobic anxiety disorder. Psychoanalytic theories have sought to explain phobias in terms of unresolved, unconscious conflicts that are symbolically expressed. So, a phobic fear of spiders supposedly derives from repressed knowledge of the sexuality of one's parents. Difficulties of verifying these theories empirically, lack of evidence for the efficacy of psychoanalytical treatment of phobias, and downright modern scepticism, have tended to result in these theoretical approaches becoming eclipsed. More weight is now given to learning theories which hypothesise that phobias develop when an experience (which may be observed or directly experienced) is accompanied or followed by extreme fear. Thus, the individual in future seeks to avoid the situation or stimulus that is associated with the fear and a phobia is the result. For instance, being in an elevator that breaks down may provoke a feeling of panic, and that experience becomes generalised to fear of going in all lifts, and perhaps beyond that to confinement in small spaces. Social workers may find themselves attempting to support people who experience phobic anxiety. The type of help that is effective has to be matched to the form of phobia, though there is evidence for the generic effectiveness of cognitive-behavioural methods:

- *Agoraphobia.* This involves a persistent and irrational fear of places from which it is difficult to exit, the difficulty may be physical or it may be socially awkward. This can include confined spaces, such as the example given above of the elevator, it may be crowded locations such as a sports event or large party, or it could be travel to a distant destination such that the person feels they cannot return home easily. Agoraphobia can lead to increasing dependency on other people for support in going about their daily lives, and they may become progressively confined to home to avoid panic-inducing situations. Social workers may be able to offer cognitive behavioural techniques such as teaching relaxation techniques and graded exposure to panic-inducing situations; this graduated exposure may initially be through imagination, or actual 'in vivo' exposure.

- *Social phobia.* This has similarities to agoraphobia but is specific to avoidance of situations that the person believes may lead to catastrophic humiliation or embarrassment; for instance, in giving a public presentation or in making a social gaffe at an event. This goes beyond 'normal' anticipatory anxiety and takes the form of severely limiting the life opportunities of the individual. Once again, cognitive behavioural techniques play a part in supporting the person to learn to face these situations and develop more realistic thoughts about the improbability of social disaster.

- *Specific phobias.* These are phobias that are targeted on specific objects or situations and include particular animals such as spiders, objects such as knives or blood, or situations such as darkness, heights or driving a motor vehicle. Very often these specific phobias are learned in childhood, although they can develop in later life in the context of stressful events. These phobias, if treated at all, are likely to be referred to a clinical psychologist, but a social worker conversant with cognitive–behavioural techniques should again be able to offer help with relaxation methods, graduated exposure and other CBT techniques.

Some people are afflicted by episodes of severe anxiety that can last for up to twenty or thirty minutes. These panic attacks – or 'panic disorder' – are qualitatively very different again from the experience of 'normal' anxiety, such that the person is fearful that they might be dying as the sensation can be accompanied by heart palpitations, difficulties in breathing and sensations of weakness in limbs. When a person experiences panic attacks without warning and in public places, this can lead to general avoidance of situations where panic may be experienced and can be the basis for the development of phobias such as agoraphobia. Again, cognitive–behavioural techniques can be helpful. With regard to all anxiety disorders, where the person presents to or are referred to a doctor, the first line of medical treatment may be the prescription of antidepressant medication or benzodiazepines (McIntosh et al., 2004).

Obsessive compulsive disorder (OCD)

Another area of difficult in people's lives that is associated with raised levels of anxiety are compulsions to repeat behaviours, or the obsessive intrusion of repetitive thoughts, that constrain their capacity to lead their lives as they would wish. The forms taken by these compulsions are variable but some are more common than others; for instance, compulsive hand washing, checking that electrical appliances are switched off, or returning home to ensure that doors and windows are locked. These behaviours may be repeated to the extent that they cannot hold down jobs because completion of the rituals takes several hours. Physical problems may develop; for example, ritualised hand washing can lead to painful skin lesions. Many of us are able to empathise to a degree with obsessive behaviours or thoughts because we can remember transient stages in childhood where we would not tread on the cracks between paving slabs or had compulsions to count objects or place them in order. Where these compulsions become dominant in someone's life, they often are able to acknowledge the irrationality of their actions or thought, while at the same time being unable to modify their behaviour. Similarly, they may have a rationalisation for their behaviour – for example, hand washing is important because it reduces risk of transmitting disease – whilst also knowing that the extent of the behaviour is unwarranted. In most cases though the person submits to the compulsion because they feel it will make their anxiety manageable, though with the concomitant distress that they know their actions are irrational. Sometimes the obsession can seem to have a symbolic function; for instance, the author worked with a woman whose compulsive hand washing seemed to intensify with the guilt feelings she felt after she had sought the accommodation of her husband – who had Alzheimer's disease – in residential accommodation. However, such interpretations seem of little help in supporting people to modify their behaviour and can be a form of blaming the individual. As with other anxiety-related problems, CBT is more likely to be helpful. It is also increasingly suspected that OCD is associated with co-existing depression, and in such instances the most productive interventions are those which ameliorate the depression (Abramowitz 2004).

Severe stress – post-traumatic stress disorder

Although it may be self-evident that after a traumatic event people may experience severe stress reactions, it has only been more recently that practitioners in the mental health field have recognised that it may be months or years before the problems caused by exposure to trauma are reported. Historically, attention has been focused primarily on combatants in war zones who develop severe reactions to their experiences, and the attempts to provide psychological support to the sufferers of 'shell shock' or 'battle fatigue'. Indeed, the development of psychological treatments for soldiers has been an important impetus in the development of group therapies and also therapeutic communities (Foulkes 1983).

Latterly, this attention has been broadened to more generic notions of trauma, and the psychological reactions that follow. This is an important area for social work because post-traumatic stress disorder (PTSD) may be a consequence of a number of the social problems routinely dealt with by social workers. PTSD affects both children and adults, so can be a consequence of child abuse, including sexual abuse, and situations in which the individual is subject to actual or threatened violence, such as domestic abuse. PTSD can result from any event that is of a highly threatening or potentially catastrophic nature, although not usually from the more common adverse life events such as loss of employment, onset of illness, or relationship breakdown (National Collaborating Centre for Mental Health 2005b).

PTSD can manifest itself in a number of ways, including:

- re-experiencing – having flashbacks, intrusive thoughts, sensations or recurring nightmares where the events that are so distressing are repeated. Children may feel compelled to continuously play-act the situation that has traumatised them;

- avoidance – individuals may take extreme steps to avoid the person, situation or location resembling or associated with the trauma;

- hyperarousal – an exaggerated level of sensitivity, being startled by events, sleep interruption and problems of concentration;

- emotional numbing – feeling disassociated from events, lacking pleasure in response to activities that were previously enjoyed, unable to respond emotionally to events;

- depression;

- drugs and alcohol abuse;

- anger;

- unexplained physical symptoms.

People with PTSD often are known to agencies because of problems, such as substance misuse or making suicide attempts, that are not identified with PTSD until a careful history is compiled which indicates that the presenting problems may be linked to events in the person's earlier history. In these situations it may be necessary to attend to the primary presenting problem, such as substance abuse, before addressing the PTSD. Where the person being assessed is a child, it may be the parent or other care-givers who are able to identify changes in behaviour such as interrupted sleep patterns or avoidance behaviours. There are some service user groups where there are higher probabilities of individuals developing PTSD, including children who have been abused, and refugees or asylum seekers. Research by the author and a colleague found that men who had been sexually abused as boys reported levels of suicidal thinking which were ten times those of non-abused men (O'Leary and Gould 2008).

Social workers have a role in assessing individuals for PTSD. They are also well placed to refer them for clinical help, to self-help groups or support groups, and where they are aware of high levels of need in their agency's catchment area, they may take a lead in creating such groups. Some survivors of trauma describe these kinds of support as the most important factors in their roads to recovery. Of course, where the circumstances generating PTSD are still present – for instance, an individual living in an abusive domestic situation, or a child or young person being abused by a care-giver – then statutory and agency procedures should be followed as a priority to protect that individual.

Research shows that there is individual variability in responses to traumatic events, and that PTSD may be a consequence for around 30 per cent of people exposed to severe trauma, though for some traumas such as rape the percentages are much higher. Where social workers are called in to support people after humanitarian disasters such as floods, or after an incident such as a terrorist attack, most people will experience short-term distress and obviously should be offered whatever practical and emotional support is appropriate and acceptable. Contrary to perceptions that are widespread amongst practitioners, there is no persuasive evidence that single-session debriefing sessions following a traumatic event are of benefit (Rose et al., 2004). Only a minority are at risk of developing PTSD. Guidance based on the research evidence therefore suggests following up people a month or so after the event to see whether specific intervention for PTSD is warranted.

The current evidence-base suggests that the most effective psychosocial intervention for PTSD is CBT focused on the traumatic event or events (National Collaborating Centre for Mental Health 2005b). Before a structured process of CBT can begin it may be necessary to spend some sessions developing a trusting relationship with the person so that they can begin to disclose or describe the traumatic events. We have considered above the basic model of CBT that emerged from Beck's work on depression. Trauma-focused CBT uses the same approach but focuses on the distorted and self-defeating thoughts that an individual experiences that are associated with the identified traumatic event (Blanchard and Hickling 2004). For example, this may include the person feeling responsible for the event that befell them, such as rape, or guilt for surviving and failing to save others that were victims of an event such as fire or terrorist attack. They may experience the recurring memories of the event as beyond their control, and have exaggerated and unrealistic fears that the same catastrophe will re-occur. The role of the therapist is to support the person to have more realistic thoughts about the circumstances of the trauma, and proportionate expectations about the risks they run in their everyday lives.

Activity 5.2 Social work interventions for mood disorders

Select any one of the mood disorders discussed above and identify what role a social worker can play in supporting a person living with the disorder and their family. Give particular consideration to approaches that address recovery and social inclusion.

Key points

- Depression is a persistent absence of positive affect and often associated with social and economic adversity, such as unemployment or poor housing. Individuals who are prone to depression often report ways of thinking that are self-defeating, and cognitive behavioural therapies can be helpful in developing more realistic and flexible ways of thinking.

- 'Post-natal blues' are common following childbirth and usually these feelings are transient, but some women are susceptible to post-natal depression. A very few experience puerperal psychosis and in these situations risk to the newborn child and any siblings need to be assessed.

- Manic episodes associated with bipolar disorder can be very disruptive to the lives of sufferers. Social workers may be able to offer support to individuals and their families, alongside medical intervention.

- For some individuals overwhelming feelings of anxiety or panic can become associated with specific situations, giving rise to phobias, or chronic avoidance of anxiety-provoking situations. Current evidence suggests that cognitive behaviour therapies are the most successful form of intervention.

- Individuals who experience severe trauma, including sexual abuse or domestic violence, may experience delayed, severe stress reactions. These reactions can seem inexplicable unless their connection to earlier trauma is understood.

Key reading

Brown, G. and Harris, T. (1978) *The Social Origins of Depression*, London: Tavistock.

Grant, A., Mills, J., Mulhern, R. and Short, N. (2004) *Cognitive Behavioural Therapy in Mental Health Care*, London: Sage Publications.

Sheppard, M. (1993) 'Maternal depression and child care: the significance for social work and social work research', *Adoption and Fostering*, 17(2): 10–15.

6 Mental health social work with adults: psychoses and personality disorders

By the end of this chapter you should have an understanding of:

- Debates around the nature of psychotic experience and whether having experiences such as hearing voices are necessarily catastrophic

- The nature and signs of schizophrenia and some of the psychosocial interventions that can be helpful to service users and carers

- The social implications of pharmacological interventions for schizophrenia

- Implications for social workers of working with people who have a 'dual diagnosis' – a major mental disorder as well as problematic use of drugs or alcohol

- Controversies associated with diagnoses of personality disorders and the challenge of improving access to services for people diagnosed as personality disordered.

Schizophrenia

The nature of psychotic experiences

Within clinical psychiatry a distinction is often made between 'neurosis' and 'psychosis'. A neurosis is deemed to be a mental disorder without any organic basis, where the 'patient' does not lose touch with external reality, in other words the person does not experience confusion in distinguishing between fantasies and false beliefs that are subjective and a product of illness, and objective, external reality. Accordingly, the conditions discussed in Chapter 5 such as depression and anxiety are judged to be neuroses because the individual retains 'insight' that their distress is produced by a mental health problem. This is contrasted with the psychoses, which are characterised as more severe disorders where there is an inability on the part of the person to distinguish between external reality and phenomena that are mentally produced as a result of the mental disorder. The most common psychosis is schizophrenia, though there are others such as persistent delusional disorder, induced delusional disorder and schizoaffective disorder. Conventionally, a distinction is made between the kinds of psychotic experiences that a person reports, and it is helpful for social workers to understand the basic terminology that is used in describing psychotic phenomena:

Chapter 5

A d*elusion* is a fixed and unshakeable belief that is held despite any evidence produced to the contrary, and that is not explicable in terms of the person's social milieu; for instance, it is not derived from and explicable in terms of their cultural or religious background. This is not to say that delusions do not reflect the preoccupations of someone's culture. For example, in developed countries they may have a flavour of science fiction, perhaps the unshakeable belief that a partner or child is really an alien or robot.

A *hallucination* is a sensory perception that arises in the absence of any objective external stimulation, and is experienced by the person as real and beyond their control. A hallucination might relate to any of the senses, so it might be a smell (perhaps the person believes they can smell gas and are choking), it might be a taste (food tastes strange and the person deduces they are being poisoned), visual (though this most often arises in the context of an organic disease) and, most commonly, is heard – usually in the form of voices.

As we shall see, it is important to grasp what is meant by the terminology of psychotic experiences to understand what is being discussed in relation to schizophrenia and other psychotic conditions. It is particularly important to be aware that what is being described are mental phenomena that are not consciously produced and controlled by the person, so talking internally to ourselves to coach ourselves to perform a task better, or singing a favourite song inside our heads, do not come within the meaning of psychotic experiences, nor do religious experiences – for example, 'speaking in tongues' – that would be deemed explicable within the religious community to which the person belongs. This is why it is so important for social workers to demonstrate cultural competence, to be able to assess behaviour within the cultural context within which experience arises. This may lead us to respond with some caution to the oft-quoted words of the American sceptic about psychiatry, Thomas Szasz (1971):

If you talk to God, you are praying. If God talks to you, you have schizophrenia.

Like Mr Salter in Evelyn Waugh's novel *Scoop*, we might say, 'Up to a point, Lord Copper'; it really depends on whether someone belongs to a faith in which hearing God speaking to you is deemed to be unremarkable. There is a growing body of research that demonstrates that the distinction between psychotic and non-psychotic experience is not as straightforward and clear-cut as suggested by conventional psychiatric textbooks. Hallucinations and delusions may be experienced by people experiencing extreme stress or deprived of sleep for long periods of time, and are also well-recognised symptoms of taking some illicit drugs, particularly hallucinogenics. People who are bereaved frequently describe as 'real' the experiences of hearing the voice of someone who has died or catching the smell of a scent associated with the deceased person. Some commentators are concerned that the medical model of schizophrenia as a disease entity imparts to professionals a very pessimistic set of expectations of the prognosis for the person diagnosed as schizophrenic. Recognising that psychotic-like experiences are quite pervasive within the wider population helps to normalise these experiences and, in the word of Williams, 'decatastrophises' the assumptions of professionals about those conditions that are categorised as the psychoses (Williams 2002). There are also service user groups (for example the Hearing Voices Network) which are seeking to reframe their relationship to delusional and hallucinatory experiences, particularly hearing voices, so as to be something that can be lived with, and can even be empowering.

Signs of schizophrenia

It could be argued that schizophrenia is the most misunderstood and stigmatising of all diagnoses in psychiatry. This is due in part to the debates that have ensued within the mental health community about the validity and reliability of the diagnosis; schizophrenia has been the focus of much of the disputation around anti-psychiatry, with critics such as Laing (1965) and Szasz (1971) using schizophrenia as the exemplar for their criticisms of the epistemological status of mental illness. In fact it is debatable whether many of the individuals that Laing described in his case studies met the criteria which would usually be required for a diagnosis of schizophrenia, but instead were people who had other kinds of psychological distress (Sedgwick 1972).

Prejudice is also a product of misunderstandings that are culturally reproduced by journalism, cinema and literature which in turn shape the public's (mis)understanding. The term 'schizophrenia' was first coined by Bleuler in 1908, from the Ancient Greek meaning 'splitting of the mind'. This seems to have contributed to the popular misconception that schizophrenia means split personality, with all the attendant stereotypes of 'Jekyll and Hyde' characters that alternate between normal and demonic behaviour. Bleuler's actual intention in coining the term was to describe the psychological fragmentation that was characteristic of the people whose mental condition he was describing.

More recently, clinicians have taken their criteria for diagnosing schizophrenia from the writing of Schneider (1959), hence the so-called 'Schneider's first rank symptoms' which have been very influential in UK mental health practice. Schneider wrote that a diagnosis of schizophrenia could be made where an underlying somatic (physical) illness had been excluded and any one of a number of abnormal experiences was present, as listed in Box 6.1 (although they did not have to be continuously present).

Box 6.1   Schneider's first rank symptoms of schizophrenia

- Auditory hallucinations:

  - running commentary (hearing an external voice commenting on what the person is saying or doing, often in a derogatory tone);

  - 'third person' hallucinations (external voices discussing or arguing about the person);

  - thought echoes (the person's thoughts are followed shortly afterwards by hearing an external voice repeating them).

- Delusions of thought control:

  - thought withdrawal (having the experience that thoughts are being 'sucked out' leaving the mind empty);

  - thought insertion (having the experience that someone else is transmitting their thoughts into your brain);

  - thought broadcasting (the feeling that private thoughts cannot be contained but are broadcast to other people).

- Delusions of control (passivity phenomena):

  - somatic passivity (the person experiences their bodily sensations as being controlled by an external force);

  - passivity of affect, impulses and volition (the person's feelings, wishes and actions are controlled by an external force).

- Delusional perception (feeling that everyday external events have some special meaning or significance).

When a person is experiencing one or more of these first rank symptoms, they may be said to be acutely unwell, or sometimes this will be described as being 'floridly' unwell. Many people who are sub-sequently diagnosed as being schizophrenic do not have these experiences continuously, they may be episodic, lasting weeks or months, and alternate with periods when the psychotic thoughts have abated. However, when these thoughts have subsided, the person may be left with so-called negative symptoms, feelings of emotional flatness and lethargy which make it difficult for them to maintain their motivation for activities of daily living such as self-care and work. They may find it difficult to respond spontaneously to social interactions and seem flat and apathetic in their relationships. These may be referred to as 'negative' or 'secondary' symptoms.

The onset of schizophrenia is often not sudden but may emerge over months or even years. This is often referred to as 'insidious onset'; a person may have led a successful life in terms of educational and occupational achievement but slowly their personality seems to change as they become more pre-occupied, withdrawn and uninterested in their self-care and social environment. There is no gender difference in the overall incidence rates of schizophrenia, which is around 1 per cent of the population if tightly defined according to core criteria, and around 2 per cent if more broadly defined (National Collaborating Centre for Mental Health 2003: 9). This makes it the most common of the psychoses. Despite the lack of difference between the sexes overall in incidence rates, there is a difference in the average age of onset, with women on average having developing signs of schizophrenia four to five years later than men (the average age of onset for men is 28 and, for women, 32) (Burton 2006). Mean averages disguise individual variation, and schizophrenia can begin at any age, but onset is rare in children and adolescents, or over the age of 45. The relative vulnerability of young adults is particularly relevant when we come to consider the work, later, of early intervention teams.

Epidemiological research has found that several social groups are over-represented in the rates of schizophrenia and this has led to a number of fierce debates. Overall, in the UK people of African-Caribbean origin are diagnosed with schizophrenia more than other ethnic groups and various explanations have been put forward for this, including the possibility that acute stress reactions are mistaken in non-European populations for schizophrenia, that there is inherent racism in the practice of psychiatry and bias in its diagnostic categories, or that the stress of racism triggers psychotic reactions (Harrison et al., 1988; Bhugra and Bhui 2001). In addition, studies over many years have found a statistical relationship between schizophrenia and membership of lower social classes and residence in inner-city areas (for an overview see Rogers and Pilgrim 2003). This has provoked a longstanding debate within medical sociology as to whether this supports a 'stress hypothesis', that the challenges of material adversity trigger schizophrenia, or a 'drift hypothesis', that the onset of schizophrenia is normally distributed across society, but that the impairments produced by psychosis lead individuals into a downward spiral leading to unemployment and residence in areas of social deprivation. The conclusive evidence in relation to settling these arguments remains elusive, but there is still an important overall lesson for social workers: that people who live with schizophrenia are in jeopardy of experiencing social exclusion and are in need of intervention that is relevant to the material effects of discrimination and socio-economic disadvantage.

The causes of schizophrenia remain unknown, and if schizophrenia emerges to be a term that covers a number of conditions, then the search for a single causal explanation may be futile. The elevated level of risk of schizophrenia between close family members (most strongly supported by studies of twins separately reared) indicates a genetic component. Other biological theories have focused on the dopamine hypothesis – that the individual either produces excess levels of dopamine, or that the brain's dopamine receptors are hyper-sensitive. While the evidence is inconclusive, a working hypothesis reasonably supported by evidence and one that maintains a social perspective is that schizophrenia is a disorder that is biopsychosocial in nature (National Collaborating Centre for Mental Health 2003: 10). Individuals may have an inherited vulnerability, but whether this develops into a psychotic disorder will also depend on the presence of, and susceptibility to, psychological and social stressors or trigger factors. What is now established, and is an important message for social workers, is the theory that schizophrenia is not caused by dysfunctional family relationships; in particular the Laingian notion of the 'schizophrenogenic mother' has not been validated by research. Although, as we shall see, the modification of family factors can have a positive effect on recovery and prevention of relapse, families cannot be blamed for a member developing schizophrenia.

The role of early intervention

It is very important that social workers try to imbue some optimism on the part of people diagnosed with schizophrenia and their carers. To avoid professional pessimism they should also remember the so-called 'rule of thirds': after an acute episode of psychosis about one-third of people recover and return to their previous level of functioning, about one-third improve but experience some continuing level of impairment, and roughly one-third of people experience continuing bouts of psychosis and may need periodic admissions to institutional care. So, there is not an inevitability that an episode of psychosis will be catastrophic for the individual, and recovery is very possible, though for a significant minority there will be a need to try to learn to live in ways that anticipate and manage further episodes. We will consider later in this chapter the role of psychosocial interventions in learning to cope with schizophrenia.

This should not be taken as grounds for minimising the extreme distress that the experience of schizophrenia induces in many people. In recent years epidemiological research has shown the very significant risk of suicides amongst people living with schizophrenia, estimated at a rate of 10 per cent (Brown 1997). Factors associated with elevated suicide risk include: being young, male, having an early onset of the disorder, being relatively intelligent, having insight into one's situation, being single, lacking social support, and having been recently discharged from hospital. This risk profile points strongly towards the need for early, community-based intervention to support people with the experience and management of schizophrenia.

This is further reinforced by the body of research which suggests that the individuals who receive early intervention achieve the best outcomes in terms of recovery. It has been found in a number of studies that the longer the psychosis goes untreated, the poorer the prognosis becomes (e.g., Loebel et al., 1992; McGorry et al., 1996). This finding has supported the view that new specialist services should be developed to reduce the length of time people with psychosis remain undiagnosed and untreated. Moreover, these researchers have argued that such services should offer services targeted at specialised, phase-specific intervention to service users in the early stages of psychosis to maximise their chances of recovery. Acting on this research, early intervention teams have been established in a number of countries, and there has been a commitment in the UK to establishing early intervention teams on a comprehensive basis. Typically, they accept referrals for individuals aged between 14 and 35 who are in the first three years of experiencing schizophrenia, and some may also accept work with individuals who may be showing signs of insidious onset of the condition in the hope of achieving some preventative outcomes, or ameliorating the severity of the impairment someone may have otherwise developed. The common-sense and ethical case for developing early intervention services is very strong, though as yet the evidence-base to demonstrate effectiveness is weak (National Collaborating Centre for Mental Health 2003: 139); as always the complexities for researchers of showing whether a service innovation produces measurable changes in outcomes are formidable, not least when health and social care services are continuously reorganised so that comparisons with 'normal' service configurations are impossible to pin down.

Treatments and their social implications

Although this book is aimed at social workers, and deals primarily with social and psychosocial perspectives in mental disorder, the first line of treatment for people with schizophrenia remains pharmacological. Given that social workers play a role in multidisciplinary teams in monitoring the compliance and response of individuals to medication, it is important to say something about current medical practice in prescribing drugs for schizophrenia, and how this is experienced by users of services. It was considered to be something of a miracle in the 1950s when it was found that drugs that were a by-product of the development of antihistamines for the treatment of allergies seemed to have a significant impact on the first rank symptoms of schizophrenia (Rose 2007). This first generation of antipsychotics included chlorpromazine, thioridazine, fluphenazine and haloperidol. Auditory hallucinations, hearing voices, significantly abated for some individuals even though they might not disappear completely. At least the voices sometimes became less intrusive. A further aspect of these antipsychotic drugs was that they could, as an alternative to forms taken orally, be administered by injection in slow-acting ('depot') form. This has widely been interpreted by medical historians as creating the precondition for closure of large asylums – that antipsychotic medication could be delivered on an outpatient basis.

The downside of the 'drug revolution' in schizophrenia was that the antipsychotics, also known as major tranquillisers, produced distressing side effects, and some of these were irreversible and occurred at relatively low dosage levels. These included symptoms that were very similar to those of Parkinson's disease – tremors, muscular rigidity and impairment of movement. Another distressing set of side effects are known as tardive dyskinesia – involuntary repetitive movements affecting facial muscles and extremities such as the hands. Social workers who worked in settings where the older generation of antipsychotic drugs were commonly used will have vivid memories of individuals who, even with medication to counter side effects, had significant levels of irreversible side effects such as facial tics, a shuffling gait and stereotyped behaviours such as 'pill rolling' mannerisms with the fingers. Sexual dysfunction, weight gain and sensitivity to sunlight further compounded the risks of these drugs. A more recent generation of drugs, the so-called 'atypical antipsychotics' or 'second generation antipsychotics', seem to be equally effective as the typical drugs in reducing the symptoms of schizophrenia, but without producing as many irreversible neurological side effects. At first it seemed as if the second generation drugs were also more effective in countering the acute symptoms of schizophrenia but recent trials are more equivocal. Also, the newer drugs have their own problematic side effects on metabolic processes, including weight gain and possibly increased risk of type-2 diabetes (American Diabetes Association 2004). Many service users find the side effects of both categories of drugs intolerable (Lieberman et al., 2005).

Some individuals who show no beneficial response to typical or atypical antipsychotics have come to be described in the clinical literature as 'treatment resistant' (a term which some users of services understandably find stigmatising). Usually, psychiatrists try at least two atypical antipsychotics but if there is no improvement in the person's level of psychosis, then Clozapine may be prescribed. This has been described as effective in 30–50 per cent of 'treatment-resistant cases', but it carries a risk of potentially fatal reaction in about 1 per cent of cases, and as a result regular blood checks to monitor for leucocyte counts are required. This elevated level of serious risk, and the reluctance of some individuals to undergo a regime of regular blood tests, means that Clozapine is not always appropriate or acceptable to service users.

Social workers are sometimes ambivalent about the use of powerful drugs to manage mental health problems, and their own role in the delivery of pharmacological interventions. Nevertheless, while drugs remain the first line of intervention, they are likely to remain part of the multidisciplinary approach. It should be remembered that all these drugs take several days to begin to have an effect, so any risks that have been assessed remain present during that time (and probably to a lower extent afterwards). If the social worker is the care coordinator or maintains regular contact in any other role, they could be the professional who first becomes aware that the person has stopped taking medication. There is a widely observed phenomenon in working in the field of psychosis: a frequent pattern of behaviour shown by an individual feeling relatively well after starting medication is to stop taking their pills, losing insight that they need medication, and then commence a downward spiral. Failure by professionals to register this process and take action has had negative consequences in a number of mental health-related tragedies.

Psychosocial interventions in schizophrenia

There is a danger that discussion of schizophrenia becomes too dominated by drug interventions, when the social aspects of intervention remain important. As even one of the mainstream medical psychiatric textbooks comments:

> Although under-utilised, psychosocial measures are often cost-effective and their importance in the treatment of schizophrenia should not be underestimated.
>
> (Burton 2006: 55)

Many younger people who experience schizophrenia are living with their families, and it is now well established that helping the family to understand what the person is experiencing, and how they can support them, can reduce their rates of relapse and admission to hospital. The research that underpins this approach with families is mainly British in origin. Initially it was shown that the attitude of the family ('family' in this context includes those people who have a significant emotional connection with the individual) to the person with schizophrenia could be characterised and measured as the level of 'expressed emotion', with families varying between whether they demonstrated 'high expressed emotion' or 'low expressed emotion'. As we have seen, the young person developing schizophrenia may become quite difficult to live with as they become more withdrawn, take less interest in their self-care, stop going to work or college, and may say things or behave in ways that are seen as bizarre. Other family members may believe they are acting in the person's best interests by confronting them about their behaviour, being critical of them and generally negative in their interactions with the individual. This criticality and negativity represents 'expressed emotion', and the higher the level of expressed emotion the greater the likelihood of relapse (Brown et al., 1962; Brown and Rutter 1966).

This work was taken on by others such as Leff, who devised methods of working with families that educated them about schizophrenia and, through the inculcation of understanding, moderated the level of expressed emotion they displayed (Leff et al., 1982). This in turn was shown by research to reduce the rate of relapse or readmission to hospitals of individuals – particularly during treatment and for up to fifteen months after treatment has ended improves treatment adherence and reduces the level of burden experienced by carers. The general lessons from the research seem to be that the intervention needs to be at least for six months, or alternatively at least ten sessions, it is more effective if the service user is included in the session, and it does not matter significantly whether families are worked with singly, or in groups of families, though dropout rates for group-based programmes are higher (Mari and Streiner 1999).

For some time there was a general consensus that Freudian-based forms of psychotherapy, usually referred to as psychodynamic or psychoanalytic therapies, were ineffective for schizophrenia (and indeed had not been developed to meet that need). Not least, there was concern that the focus of such therapies on powerful emotional responses to the therapist could be counter-productive, raising the stress level of the individual and hence exacerbating their level of psychosis. Some approaches to psychodynamic therapy for schizophrenia were developed but systematic reviews of the evidence for their effectiveness, including a rigorous Cochrane review (Malmberg and Fenton 2001) failed to identify evidence for their effectiveness.

More promising in recent years has been the emergence of cognitive behavioural therapies (CBTs) to help people cope better with the management of their own symptoms of schizophrenia. As we saw in the discussion of depression, CBT was originally developed as a method for intervening to modify self-defeating, depression-inducing ways of thinking. It has also more recently been introduced as an approach to working with people experiencing or prone to psychoses. Although initially targeted at the reduction of psychotic symptoms it has been extended to include a range of thoughts, feelings and behaviours that could helpfully be modified. CBT in relation to schizophrenia has been defined by Pilling et al. (2002) as a discrete psychological intervention that:

- encourages recipients to establish links between their thoughts, feelings or actions with respect to the current or past symptoms;

- allows recipients to re-evaluate their perceptions, beliefs or reasoning related to the target symptoms;

- involves at least *one* of the following: (a) monitoring of recipients' own thoughts, feelings or behaviour with respect to the symptom; (b) promotion of alternative ways of coping with the target symptom; (c) reduction of stress.

There is an emerging evidence-base for the usefulness of CBT in relation to schizophrenia, with strong evidence that it is particularly helpful with persistent symptoms. It can also help people to develop greater insight to their problems and increases the likelihood of cooperating with treatment. A systematic review of randomised trials of CBT suggests that intervention needs to last for at least six months and to include ten or more sessions (National Collaborating Centre for Mental Health 2009). When CBT is continued for more than three months there is also evidence that relapse rates are reduced. As social work training becomes more evidence-based, it is to be hoped that more practitioners will be equipped to offer CBT, and also there may be opportunities post-qualifying for developing expertise through programmes to increase access to psychological treatments.

Activity 6.1 Making an initial assessment

Mark is a 20-year-old man who has left university at the end of his first year of studies, telling friends and family that he just couldn't concentrate sufficiently to make a success of his course. He has returned to live with his parents and younger sister. Increasingly, he seems reluctant to leave his bedroom and has started to take his meals there. Mark seems to spend most of his time reading material on the Internet about the occult and has painted various esoteric symbols on his bedroom door. Any attempts by his parents or sister to encourage him out of his bedroom or to be distracted from his interests have resulted in abrupt and angry verbal responses.

You are visiting the family as the social worker in a Community Mental Health Team, and attempting to engage with Mark in dialogue about his situation. From the information provided above, what constructions could be placed upon Mark's behaviour, and what areas of his life and recent history would you wish to explore further in order to help your assessment?

The challenge of dual diagnosis

Perhaps one of the most challenging client groups that social workers will encounter are those who simultaneously experience a psychotic disorder and at the same time are problem users of drugs or alcohol, people with a so-called dual diagnosis. It has been estimated that about one-third of people who have been diagnosed with schizophrenia also use illicit substances (Wright et al., 2000). Although this has been recognised as a difficult area for services for up to twenty years in the USA and Europe, it is perceived by practitioners to be a worsening problem. Dual diagnosis does not have to refer to the co-existence of substance misuse and schizophrenia specifically, it could be another form of psychosis, but this is the most frequent combination. People with a dual diagnosis are particularly problematic for mental health services because of the chaos that frequently characterises their lifestyle – often precarious living arrangements including homelessness – and the unhelpful separation historically of services for addressing mental health problems and drug and alcohol dependency.

The reasons why an individual might have a co-existence of a mental health and dependency problem has been helpfully conceptualised by Lehman et al. (1989) as falling into four categories or sub-types:

*   mental illness is the primary problem with secondary problems of substance misuse;

*   primary substance misuse with psychiatric consequences;

*   dual primary diagnosis;

*   mental illness and substance misuse that have a common causative factor such as post-traumatic stress disorder or sexual abuse.

A social assessment prepared by a social worker, or multidisciplinary assessment to which a social worker contributes the social content, can be helpful in identifying which of these four categories is relevant to the particular case. In turn this is helpful in disentangling what should be the main focus of intervention. A not uncommon scenario is the young person who begins to have abnormal experiences, perhaps hearing voices or developing paranoid ideas, who finds that smoking cannabis or drinking alcohol excessively dulls the distressing experiences. The second category, the provocation of psychiatric consequences by substance abuse, can take various forms. Sustained abuse of amphetamines produces psychotic reactions that are indistinguishable from schizophrenia, but which remit when the person desists from taking amphetamines. There is a current public and professional anxiety about the availability of strong forms of cannabis (particularly 'skunk') and the onset of schizophrenia, that is, that this is not self-medication as in the first category, but that the cannabis plays a causative role in the schizophrenia. The clarity of this debate has not been helped by the history of psychiatric diagnoses such as 'ganja psychosis' that seemed to be imbued with racist assumptions about the sectors of the population to which it applied – young, black men – and those to whom it was never applied – such as white, middle-class students who smoked 'dope'.

The third category in Lehman et al.'s typology is where the two conditions of substance misuse and mental health disorder are of equal significance. Finally, both mental disorder and substance misuse may be produced by a third factor such as post-traumatic stress or sexual abuse. Research has shown how men who were sexually abused as boys may develop maladaptive coping mechanisms such as alcohol abuse or drug-taking amongst other problematic behaviours (O'Leary and Gould 2008). These men also tend to be over-represented amongst the numbers diagnosed with a variety of mental health problems. Disentangling the causal relationships between abuse, substance misuse and mental disorder is highly complex and still needs further research, but there are clear implications for practitioners that such individuals need to be carefully assessed, not least to identify risk factors such as suicidal thinking (O'Leary and Gould 2008).

Individuals with dual diagnosis may need considerable amounts of practical support with housing, financial and employment difficulties, but also psychosocial help with stabilising their lives and engaging with services. Osher and Kofoed (1989) have developed a four-stage model (outlined in Box 6.2), though as with any stage-based model it has to be accepted that there will be individual variation in how people move through the stages, and periods when they go back to previous stages. As in working with Prochaska and DiClemente's (1986) well-known model, the practitioner has to be prepared to develop a relationship that is non-judgemental and positive (making a 'therapeutic alliance') and working at the individual's own rate of change.

Box 6.2   Osher and Kofoed's (1989) four-stage model for working with people living with dual diagnosis

- Stage 1: Engagement. Given the likelihood that the person will be living a chaotic existence and without a high level of motivation to engage with services, it may be necessary to engage through assertive outreach. At this early stage a priority for intervention may be to encourage the individual to adopt safer, harm-reduction methods for imbibing problem substances, be it clean syringes, avoiding drinking toxic substances or using a water vapouriser to reduce the effects of smoking on the lungs.

- Stage 2: Building motivation. This may include individual and family education so that those involved are more informed about the problems and their possible solutions. Motivational interviewing, now commonly introduced to social workers undertaking qualifying studies, helps the person to address their ambivalence about reducing their substance misuse. The practitioner works with the service user to identify when they are ready to move on from feeling ambivalent to tackling their substance problem.

- Stage 3: Active engagement. This is where the practitioner works with the person with dual diagnosis to identify targets for intervention, and selects the method to achieve change. The social environment is significant in this as the person who abuses substances is likely to have developed social networks of people with similar habits, and part of the focus of inter-vention may include developing new social outlets where peer pressure is removed or at least reduced. This is easier said than done as, even working on inpatient units, drug and alcohol misuse is all-pervasive.

- Stage 4: Relapse prevention. This is the stage beyond the modification of behaviour relating to substance abuse, and is the development of strategies for avoiding relapse. Rather than one solution this is likely to involve the development of a repertoire of strategies including social skills training, cognitive strategies and lifestyle changes. Hopefully, these give the person choices as to how they will deal with situations that produce the kinds of stress or temptation that previously have led to harmful use of substances.

Working with people with personality disorders

This chapter concludes by looking at the personality disorders, the controversial status of these diagnoses, and the challenges of working with people described as having a personality disorder. We have considered the public stigma of the label of schizophrenia, but personality disorders are possibly the most stigmatising labels amongst professional mental health workers themselves. They tend to be people who professionals experience as difficult to relate to, sometimes disruptive and self-destructive in their behaviour, and it has been difficult to establish that medical or social interventions are effec-tive. Consequently, psychiatrists and other mental health workers have striven to divert them away from mental health services, either towards the criminal justice system or leaving them without referral to any services or support. As an official report that included the views of people with personality disorders stated:

> No mental disorder carries a greater stigma than the diagnosis 'Personality Disorder', and those diagnosed can feel labelled by professionals as well as by society. There was a strong feeling that many professionals did not understand the diagnosis, and often equated it with untreatability. Those with personality disorder have been described as '*the patients psychiatrists dislike*', and many reported being called time-wasters, difficult, manipulative, bed-wasters or attention-seeking.
>
> (National Institute for Mental Health England 2003: 20)

By coincidence, the modern history of the concept of personality disorder originates, as with schizophrenia, with the writing of Kurt Schneider, who described 'psychopathic personalities' in his textbook of the same name (1923). Psychopathic personality disorder was further elaborated and sub-categorised by Henderson (1939) who included in his typology the 'creative psychopath', people who find a creative and socially respectable niche for their aggressive urges. He cited Lawrence of Arabia as an example but many people would be tempted to substitute the political leader they most dislike. Psychopathic personality disorder continued to be used as a mainstream diagnosis although there was always controversy that this had no validity as a medical diagnosis, and was a catch all for people who society found inexplicably hostile and disruptive ('they must be mad to have done that') (Prins 1980). Not least there was a fundamental circularity to the diagnosis; psychopathy was defined as abnormally aggressive and antisocial behaviour and people were diagnosed as psychopathic by their antisocial and criminal behaviour, but the diagnosis had no 'symptoms' other than that same behaviour. This was reified by the 1983 Mental Health Act which included psychopathic disorder as a mental illness that could warrant compulsory detention. The conceptual problems of the diagnostic approach to personality disorder is well summed up in the NICE treatment guideline for antisocial personality disorder:

> The *DSM-IV* definition has other major limitations including problems of overlap between the differing personality disorder diagnoses, heterogeneity among individuals with the same diag-nosis, inadequate capture of personality psychopathology and growing evidence in favour of a dimensional rather than a categorical system of classification.
>
> (NICE 2008: 15)

To try to deal with these problems, the diagnosis has become more elaborated and refined, reflecting two theoretical approaches to the development of unusual personality types. On the one hand, psychoanalytical commentators have described personality disorders in terms of disruptions to attachments in early childhood which interrupt and distort the formation of ego defence mechanisms. Cognitively oriented writers similarly emphasise early trauma or unstable relationships, but their explanatory framework emphasises the development of 'cognitive schemas' or ways of processing information in ways that seek to maintain a sense of self-consistency that are maladaptive. It may be that these approaches are ultimately not mutually exclusive. *ICD-10* and *DSM-IV* categorise personality disorders by sub-types of personality disorder that are similar if not exactly the same. There is a danger that allocating individuals to these sub-types becomes rather like butterfly collecting – looking for exotic examples of obscure diagnoses – and demeans and reduces individuals to their label. This is particularly doubtful as an exercise as even clinicians agree that most people fall into more than one diagnostic category, or have a dual diagnosis of a personality disorder and another form of mental illness.

Some coherence and manageability is at least introduced to all this by *DSM-IV*'s clustering of per-sonality disorders into three main categories or clusters, and it is helpful for mental health social workers to have a basic understanding of the differentiations.

Cluster A:

- Paranoid personality disorder – having a pervasive distrust of others.

- Schizoid personality disorder – being detached and aloof, prone to introspection/fantasy.

- Schizotypal personality disorder – eccentric behaviour and thinking similar to schizophrenia.

Cluster B:

- Antisocial personality disorder – callous unconcern for others, impulsivity and aggression.

- Borderline personality disorder – lacking a sense of self with emotional instability and self-harm.

- Histrionic personality disorder – self-centred, attention-seeking and seeming to play a role rather than responding to situations authentically.

- Narcissistic personality disorder – grandiose and self-important and lacking in empathy.

Cluster C:

- Anxious-avoidant personality disorder – feeing socially inept or inferior and, consequently, anxious.

- Dependent personality disorder – lack of self-confidence and an excessive need to be taken care of.

- Obsessive–compulsive personality disorder/anankastic – obsessed with details, lists and order, with rigidity and humourlessness in relationships.

Some of these sub-types are so broadly defined that it may be conjectured as to where the boundary lies between supposed 'illness' and eccentricity. The prevalence rate for personality disorders has been found to be 4.4 per cent of the population in Great Britain, with higher concentrations in urban centres (Coid et al., 2006). When the occurrence of a condition is stated as being this high, it does raise questions about whether this can meaningfully be understood, particularly from the perspective of a medical model, as a disease entity. This seems to reinforce at least some of the criticisms of those who say that the label reflects normative judgements about social behaviour and is a convenient way of categorising those people who are experienced by the wider society as odd or difficult. Social workers practising in mainstream settings will be used to working with a range of service users who probably would meet clinical criteria of being personality disordered, yet they are not in contact with mental health services or formally diagnosed; social workers routinely provide services to them on the basis of their social needs.

As indicated, where a formal diagnosis of personality disorder is made this can become a rationalisation for excluding people from services, as they are assumed to be difficult and 'untreatable'. In recent years there has been an attempt to address this form of social exclusion within health and social care services by inculcating a greater sense of optimism about working with people with personality disorders, symbolised by the Department of Health report *Personality Disorder: No Longer a Diagnosis of Exclusion*

(National Institute for Mental Health England 2003). Research with service users who have been diagnosed with personality disorders has helped to establish what is so resented by them about the label:

> Some felt that a more appropriate description would be 'attachment-seeking'. They felt blamed for their condition and often sought basic acceptance and someone to listen to them. They sought to gain legitimacy rather than being told 'you're not mentally ill'. Some preferred terms such as 'emotional distress'.
>
> (National Institute for Mental Health 2003: 20)

Service users consulted for this report were clear about what they would find helpful and positive in the responses they received from services, as summarised in Box 6.3.

Box 6.3   Helpful features for personality disorder services as identified by service users

- Early interventions, before crisis point
- Specialist services, not part of general MH
- Choice from a range of treatment options
- Individually tailored care
- Therapeutic optimism and high expectations
- Develops patients' skills
- Fosters the use of creativity
- Respects strengths and weaknesses
- Good clear communication
- Accepting, reliable, consistent
- Clear and negotiated treatment contracts
- Focus on education and personal development
- Good assessment/treatment link
- Conducive environment
- Listens to feedback and has strong voice from service users

---

- Supportive peer networks

- Shared understanding of boundaries

- Appropriate follow-up and continuing care

- Involves patients as experts

- Attitude of acceptance and sympathy

- Atmosphere of 'truth and trust'

(National Institute for Mental Health England 2003: 22)

Two forms of personality disorder that are receiving particular attention for the development of evidence-based interventions, and which will be encountered by social workers practising in mental health settings, are borderline personality disorder and antisocial personality disorder. The diagnostic system *DSM-IV* defines antisocial personality disorder as a pervasive pattern of disregard for and violation of the rights of others that has been occurring in the individual since the age of 15 years, as indicated by three (or more) of seven criteria: a failure to conform to social norms; irresponsibility; deceitfulness; indifference to the welfare of others; recklessness; a failure to plan ahead; and irritability and aggressiveness (American Psychiatric Association 1994). Antisocial personality disorder is mainly diagnosed in men, and is highly prevalent in males who are imprisoned. However, it would be an over-simplification to equate antisocial personality disorder with offending as community-based studies find a preponderance of people meeting the criteria for antisocial personality disorder are living in the community. Their lives are characterised not by illegal behaviour but by a range of self-destructive and impulsive behaviours that lead to a range of poor social outcomes including unemployment, housing problems and interrupted family relationships (Paris 2003).

When the author was a practitioner in forensic settings, the accepted wisdom was that this condition began to abate as men matured beyond the age of 40, and without any effective intervention the only option was to contain and monitor them until middle age. This is now challenged by evidence showing that such individuals continue to have difficulties through the life course (Paris 2003). There is also distressing evidence that individuals with antisocial personality disorder disproportionately meet pre-mature deaths, resulting from events such as suicide, drug abuse and being the victims of interpersonal violence (Black et al., 1996).

However, there is now an evidence-base that suggests that some forms of cognitive and behavioural intervention are helpful in meeting the needs of people with antisocial personality disorder, particularly in reducing offending behaviour. Also, given that many adults with antisocial personality disorder will

Chapter 4

have demonstrated conduct disorders as children, parenting education and training programmes offer a form of preventative intervention (see Chapter 4).

For adults, the evidence for effective interventions points towards the use of cognitive behavioural therapies (Duggan et al., 2007). Some of the programmes with the most robust evidence in support of them will already be known to probation officers and others working in criminal justice systems; for example, Reasoning and Rehabilitation (Ross et al., 1988). These are structured programmes which encourage individuals to identify their reasoning styles that lead them to make poor decisions and act impulsively and antisocially, and to develop more productive strategies for problem-solving. A limitation of the evidence-base is that the main reported outcome measures are rates of re-offending, with all the problems of circularity to which we have referred. This pays no attention to the modification of personality or reduction in non-offending dysfunctional behaviour.

It should not be overlooked that many people with antisocial personality disorder also have other common mental health problems such as depression and anxiety, and dependency on alcohol or drugs. Such individuals can still benefit from the interventions that would be helpful for individuals without antisocial personality disorders, in other words they should not be denied the offer of such help.

Whereas antisocial personality disorder is primarily diagnosed in men, borderline personality disorder is more often ascribed to women with a gender ratio of 3:1 (Burton 2006: 110), though it could be that the research that finds this gender bias is based on clinical populations and reflects women's greater readiness to seek help. Community-based surveys find less gender imbalance (Moran et al., 2000). A diagnosis of borderline personality disorder is made when five from a list of criteria are demonstrated: avoidance of real or imagined abandonment, unstable and intense personal relationships, switching between idealised and negative views of others, an unstable self-image or sense of self, impulsivity in at least two areas that are self-damaging such as substance abuse, impulsive sex, dangerous driving or binge eating, suicidal or self-mutilating behaviour, marked mood instability, chronic feelings of emptiness, inappropriate anger or problems in controlling anger, and transient stress-related paranoid thinking (Mills et al., 2004: 83).

There is a consensus in the clinical and psychological literature that borderline personality disorder is often associated with developmental problems in childhood, particularly environments which are abusive or where the individual has felt that their emotions are not understood or validated. As is the state of knowledge in so much of mental health, it is not clear whether these adversities in childhood are causal, or whether the child's behaviour leads to negative and damaging experiences. Cognitive psychologists see that they have then developed schemas or 'rules for living' that are strategies for dealing with feelings produced by that lack of validation. For instance, they may avoid intimacy because they believe that anyone who got to know them at a deeper level would not love, or even like, them. More psychoanalytically orientated observers have described similar behaviours in terms of ego defence mechanisms such as 'splitting' (separating others into good or bad people on the basis of selective perception of their attributes) and 'projection' (attributing feelings that are unacceptable to oneself to others).

The most promising methods for working therapeutically with people with borderline personality disorder draw eclectically from both cognitive and psychoanalytic perspectives. For example, *cognitive analytical therapy* focuses on developing a relationship with the service user, and as emotions arise in the relationship, attempting to identify how they arise and relate to the person's underlying tendencies to inappropriately intense feelings or depersonalisation. *Dialectical behaviour therapy* is particularly formulated for helping women with borderline personality disorder who self-harm, and aims to give them social skills for dealing more effectively with stress-inducing situations while supporting them through empathy and validation of feelings. Bateman and Tyrer's (2002) review, commissioned by the National Institute for Mental Health England, of the effectiveness of different therapeutic approaches is cautiously optimistic that interventions are helpful, although it may be the generic features of approaches that are therapeutic rather than any particular approach standing out as evidence based. They identify those generic features as being that the intervention:

- is well structured;

- has attention devoted to adherence to the method;

- has a clear focus;

- is theoretically coherent to the service user and therapist;

- is relatively long term;

- is integrated with other services available to the service user;

- involves a clear treatment alliance between therapist and service user.

(Bateman and Tyrer cited NIMHE 2003: 23)

Overall then, there is a concerted effort within mental health services to turn around traditional messages of despair – that people with personality disorders are beyond help and absorb disproportionate amounts of time and resources because of their disruptive behaviour – towards accepting that these attitudes serve to socially exclude those individuals and that intervention can promote recovery. Along with continuing attempts to research interventions to establish those that are most effective, services are being developed to meet the needs of people with personality disorders. The Department of Health's encouragement to local trusts to develop specialist personality disorder teams, with relevant training in therapeutic methods for practitioners is one step in this direction (National Institute for Mental Health England 2003: 30).

Activity 6.2 Working with people with personality disorders

On the basis of what you have read in this chapter about people diagnosed with personality disorders:

- identify three or more reasons why this group of service users has traditionally been regarded as problematic or challenging by mental health services;

- suggest ways in which services can make themselves more relevant and accessible to people with personality disorders;

- identify those forms of intervention which are evidence based in relation to personality disorders, noting the specific forms of personality disorder for which they are effective.

Key points

- A psychotic experience is one where the individual is unable to distinguish between external reality and internal mental phenomena such as delusions, hallucinations or false beliefs. However, research suggests that the distinction between psychotic and non-psychotic experiences is not unproblematic, as many 'normal' individuals also report these experiences.

- Schizophrenia is diagnosed when an underlying physical illness has been excluded and an individual reports the experience of auditory hallucination, delusions of thought control, delusions of passivity, or a delusional perception of special significance of external events.

- There is a growing body of evidence that early intervention for schizophrenia achieves the best outcomes in terms of recovery.

- Although drug treatments are conventionally used as the first line of treatment, there is evidence for the helpfulness of psychosocial interventions including family education programmes and cognitive behaviour therapies.

- Individuals with a dual diagnosis of schizophrenia and substance misuse present particular challenges to service providers but social workers can offer psychosocial help to stabilise their lives.

- Some progress is being made in developing psychological interventions, including approaches relevant to antisocial and borderline personality disorders.

- Recognising that a diagnosis of personality disorder has often been a basis for excluding people from services, guidelines have been developed to make local services more accessible and relevant.

Key reading

Harris, N., Williams, S and Bradshaw, T. (eds) (2002) *Psychosocial Interventions for People with Schizophrenia*, Basingstoke: Palgrave Macmillan.

National Collaborating Centre for Mental Health (2009) *Schizophrenia. Full national clinical guideline on core interventions for primary and secondary care (update).* London: The British Psychological Society and Gaskell.

National Institute for Mental Health (England) (2003) *Personality Disorder: No longer a diagnosis of exclusion*, London: Department of Health.

7 Mental health social work with older people

By the end of this chapter you should have an understanding of:

- The negative stereotyping of older people as a social and economic burden, and implications of this for our view of mental health in old age

- Signs of dementia and the main diagnostic categories or types of dementia

- How to recognise dementia and approaches to assessing the social needs of people living with dementia

- The importance within dementia care of Kitwood's concept of person-centred care

- The relative evidence of effectiveness for psychosocial interventions in dementia care

- The importance of end of life care for people with dementia

- The prevalence of depression as a mental health issue in older age and its significance for social care services

- The importance of giving attention to the needs of individuals who care for older people with mental health problems

- The needs of older people with longstanding mental health problems.

Ageing and mental health stereotypes

Old age and older people are frequently characterised by negative imagery. Even a recent social work periodical, from which more sensitivity might be expected, recently carried the headline 'dementia time bomb'. The concept of a time bomb seems to be the most beloved cliché of journalists and feature writers who commonly refer to changing population trends as inherently problematic for society. Phillipson (1982) has characterised this as 'the crisis of old age'. After the Second World War and until the 1960s, policy discourse about old age was dominated by the role of the welfare state to provide security beyond retirement. The 1970s and 1980s saw a fiscal crisis of the welfare state, its expansion compromised by global recession and panics about the affordability of welfare. From the 1990s onwards we have seen residualisation of the welfare state in providing for old age with consequent scapegoating of older people as a drain on society.

The clear implication is that older people are a problem, a burden, and make little economic or social contribution. Sometimes these popular stereotypes have been reinforced by academic sociological and psychological theories which imply that decline and loss of function are inevitable, such as some psychosocial theories of the life-cycle which stress disengagement from social interaction in later life as 'normal' (e.g., Cumming and Henry 1961; Erikson 1977). Yet this is at odds with any objective appraisal of the role that older people play in social life. They are the backbone of voluntary organisations and in the professions that permit practitioners to continue working beyond the statutory retirement age – such as law and medicine – individuals may be active into their eighth decade. Statistics for participation rates in adult learning (Age Concern 2007) show that many older individuals continue to be active learners in the later phases of their lives. Demographic changes in developed countries, with longer age expectancy and declining birth rates, are themselves leading to reappraisal of the nature of old age with greater flexibilities for people to remain active in the workplace until later in life.

It is also the case that, despite media portrayals, most people retain their psychological well-being throughout their lives. At the same time, it is also important for social workers to be aware that increasing age does bring with it greater risk of experiencing certain mental health problems. Some of these are strongly correlated with (but not synonymous with) the physiological ageing process, such as the dementias. Other conditions, notably depression and anxiety, are not uncommon with old age and may be associated with greater vulnerabilities to mental distress if ageing is accompanied by loss of social networks and stimulation. At the same time, living to an older age does not preclude the (relatively rare) development of conditions such as schizophrenia normally associated with onset at a younger age. We need to steer a balanced course between pathologising older people, while at the same time being informed about mental distress that may be associated with longevity. Social workers need to be aware of the main indicators of mental distress (and how they can sometimes be confused with reversible physiological conditions) and to have knowledge of methods of intervention for which there is evidence that they offer benefit to users of services and their carers.

Dementia – signs and types

> Dementia is a term for a range of progressive, terminal organic brain diseases.
>
> (National Audit Office 2007: 5)

An authoritative report produced by the Alzheimer's Society in 2007, the *Dementia UK* report (Alzheimer's Society 2007), estimated that there are 683,597 people living with dementia in the UK. Increasing longevity means that incidence will rise, unless there are treatment breakthroughs, reaching over 940,110 by 2021. Dementia is estimated to account for 10 per cent of deaths of men aged over 65, and 15 per cent of women aged over 65 (Alzheimer's Society 2007), although many more people will die of other causes while living with dementia. These figures have to be treated as estimates given that frequently there are failures to diagnose dementia until it is well advanced, if at all. The main risk factor for dementia is age, with 12.2 per cent of people living with dementia at the age of 82 (Alzheimer's Society 2007). The correlation between dementia and age tends to render less visible others who are living with dementia. Thus, people with learning difficulties, particularly those living with conditions that carry cardiovascular complications such as Down's syndrome, have higher susceptibility to dementia. Also, there are estimated to be more than 15,000 people in England who are aged under 65 living with dementia (Alzheimer's Society 2007). Such people, because of their relatively sound physical health, are also likely to live longer with the condition. Life expectancy with dementia varies significantly, the average time between diagnosis and death being eleven to twelve years, but this can extend to twenty years depending on whether diagnosis is made early and the underlying physical health of the individual.

Box 7.1   Common types of dementia

- Alzheimer's disease (AD). Accounts for roughly 60 per cent of cases, causes unknown but associated with various pathological changes in the brain. Usually a global and progressive accumulation of symptoms, but memory loss in earlier stages is common with later mood changes and behavioural problems. Begins insidiously with gradual changes in cognition, particularly loss of short-term memory.

- Vascular dementia (VaD). Accounts for 10–20 per cent of cases, if mixed AD and VaD is included. This is due to stroke disease or poor cerebral circulation. In contrast to AD, VaD tends to have a sudden onset and stepwise progression. Symptoms tend to depend on the location of the infarcts (tissue death due to sudden loss of blood supply) in the brain but mood and behavioural changes are common.

- Dementia with Lewy bodies (DLB). A recently discovered form of dementia that accounts for around 20 per cent of cases. Previously mistaken for dementia caused by Parkinson's disease and, as the causes of DLB are still unclear, it is possible that the two conditions are part of a spectrum. Characterised by fluctuating cognitive impairments, confusional episodes and visual hallucinations. Can be mistaken for Parkinson's disease because of frequent occurrence of muscular rigidity, falls and resting tremor.

- There are many other types and causes of dementia including frontotemporal dementia (the commonest form of young onset dementia), degenerative diseases such as Parkinson's disease, Huntingdon's disease, Creutzfeldt-Jakob disease (CJD), HIV-AIDs, and various metabolic disorders including alcohol-related dementia.

Conventionally, a distinction is made between young-onset dementia which commences before the individual reaches the age of 65 (previously called 'pre-senile dementia') and late-onset dementia, referring to those who develop the condition after the age of 65. This distinction continues to be employed in psychiatry as the characteristics and etiology of people with dementia vary between younger and older people, and individuals at different stages in their life course may need different forms of support. This has led in some areas to the establishment of local specialist young-onset dementia services.

There are numerous conditions that cause the symptoms of dementia. The most common is Alzheimer's disease (AD), which accounts for roughly 60 per cent of all cases (Alzheimer's Society 2007: xiv). AD, in its earlier stages presents itself with loss of memory, especially for retaining new information (sometimes referred to as loss of short-term memory). This relates to those areas of the brain (the medial temporal lobe and the hippocampus) which are the main sites of change. As the condition develops and affects other parts of the brain, then other functions begin to be affected such as language, praxis and executive function. In turn these changes are reflected in a range of behavioural responses that may include agitation, disinhibition (sometimes sexual), delusions and hallucinations, wandering, incontinence, breakdown of rhythms of sleeping and waking and altered eating habits. The occurrence and presentation of these behavioural changes are unique to the individual, may not be exhibited by everyone, and are variable in their order of presentation.

It is usually the cumulative effect of these behavioural changes that causes great distress to both the individuals affected and their carers, often more so than the development of cognitive impairments.

As impairment increases, independence tends to diminish with problems of self-care including dressing, washing, eating and toileting. Research suggests that these behaviours that challenge are also the most significant factors in determining whether individuals continue to live in the community or enter residential care (Bianchetti et al., 1995). Sometimes behavioural changes can present themselves earlier than memory impairment, but this is unusual and may indicate other cause for the dementia. People with AD may experience short periods when their condition plateaus but the progress of the condition is fairly continuous.

Cerebrovascular disease is a common cause of dementia (referred to as vascular dementia (VaD)). This can present itself after an individual has a 'stroke' (an acute vascular event) or it can develop more insidiously as a result of insidious vascular problems with the gradual onset of problems of attention and decision-making. As with AD, behaviours that challenge are common, and individuals may become depressed and apathetic. VaD is less continuous and persistent than AD in its progress as the underlying vascular problems might stabilise. Alternatively, a new vascular event or stroke can precipitate a sudden deterioration in function. The difference between AD and VaD is sometimes represented graphically with AD represented by a continuous downward line, and VaD by a 'spiky' line of peaks and troughs, albeit with an overall downward trend.

A more recently discovered condition is dementia with Lewy bodies (DLB), accounting for a further 15–20 per cent of occurrences (McKeith and Fairbairn 2001). This was discovered by a Newcastle-based group of psychiatrists specialising in old age who realised that a sub-group of their patients had a distinctive set of symptoms, some of which had previously been mistaken for Parkinson's disease. People with DLB may manifest the motor problems associated with Parkinsonism such as tremors and muscular rigidity (though 25 per cent do not develop these features), but also experience cognitive disturbance, visual hallucinations, falls, disturbances of consciousness and rapid eye movement sleep behaviour disorder (McKeith et al., 2005). The course of DLB can fluctuate dramatically over time, though the overall trend is one of deterioration, and the combination of cognitive and motor problems produces significant problems for the individual.

Increasingly, it has been recognised that individuals may have more than one cause of their dementia, that it can be of mixed-type, for instance AD with VaD, and a large autopsy-based study in the UK found that for older people at death mixed pathology was the most common finding (Medical Research Council 2001).

For people with young-onset dementia, a common cause is frontotemporal dementia, but other causes exist including degenerative diseases such as Huntingdon's disease, Creutzfeldt-Jakob disease (CJD), HIV-AIDs and various metabolic disorders including alcohol-related dementia. Dementia also occurs in 30–70 per cent of people with Parkinson's disease. For clinicians, the distinction between Parkinson's disease and DLB can be difficult to make, and is made on the basis of the chronology of the appearance of symptoms. If dementia precedes the occurrence of motor problems, or is detected within twelve months of them, then DLB is diagnosed (McKeith et al., 2005).

For the social worker it is helpful to know some of these distinct traits of conditions underlying the signs of dementia but, overall, the rate of cognitive decline is noticeably consistent across the three principal types of dementia, measured as 3–4 points per year using the Mini Mental State Examination (National Collaborating Centre for Mental Health 2006a: 70). Also, for all people with dementia there are increased physical health risks. Not surprisingly, given the nature of the underlying pathology, people with VaD are more susceptible to dying from cardiovascular and cerebrovascular disease. Lack of attention to self-care and diet, along with decreasing mobility make people with dementia more susceptible to other illnesses. Weight loss and nutritional deficiencies are common problems. It is not surprising that, as these inter-related difficulties develop for the individual, there will be multiple contacts with health and social services. Over its course, dementia impacts on so-called activities of daily living, initially in terms of shopping, maintaining a domestic routine and self-care, but later also mobility, toileting and verbal communication. All these factors combine to produce increasing challenges to independence and greater reliance on family, friends, neighbours and community-based services.

Although dementia is predominantly characterised as an organic, irreversible and terminal condition, in the last decade there have been important contributions which have focused on dementia as a psychosocial condition. This is not to deny that ageing can be associated with biological conditions in the brain, but seek to balance biological reductionism with an understanding that the way in which physiological processes are experienced is highly mediated by sociological and psychological aspects of the individual's personal biography. For example, Cheston and Bender (1999), who are both psychologists, have argued that social, psychological and organic factors interact in a dialectical fashion so that dementia cannot be fully understood as an organic illness any more than it could be simply as a social or psychological problem. For Cheston and Bender the concept which connects these domains of the biological, social and psychological is the notion of loss of social role. As individuals progressively become regarded as unable to function responsibly, and their lives become taken over by others, so loss of role and status occurs. Yet it is our social role, our sense of who we are and the contribution we make to our family, community and wider society that acts as the buffer against personal disintegration. Cheston and Benders' arguments in relation to the social construction of dementia are closely related to Kitwood and others' theory of 'person-centred care' and will be returned to later in the chapter. For the social worker these perspectives are important because they point to areas of social functioning which are important to assess at an early stage of contact with a person who may have dementia; they also counter more pessimistic approaches that dementia is irreversible. If dementia is mediated by factors located within the social environment, then these may be amenable to intervention and amelioration.

Recognising and assessing dementia

An obstacle to progressive practice with people living with dementia has been the continuing use of language which is both pejorative and misleading. Thus, we often hear people being described as 'senile', but this has no clinical status and is a term which is labelling and stigmatising and should not be used in professional discourse. 'Elderly mentally infirm' similarly has no diagnostic status and is a term originally formulated by civil servants as a euphemistic term to refer to services for people living with dementia: 'E.M.I' continues to be a descriptor applied to care homes and day services but is questionably discriminatory by association with poor institutional practices.

'Confusion' in particular is a term that can be used loosely and imprecisely by workers or carers as synonymous with dementia. The term's use should be restricted to the delirium produced by underlying physiological problems, which if appropriately treated are often reversible (McKeith and Fairbairn 2001). If someone suddenly begins to exhibit dementia-like signs such as forgetfulness, but this is accompanied by hallucinations, misinterpreting of events or clouding of consciousness, this may indicate the presence of delirium. Confusion may be the result of underlying physical illness such as urinary or chest infections, congenital heart failure, hypothyroidism, diabetes, vitamin B12 deficiency or the side effects of drugs (older people can be more susceptible to side effects of prescribed drugs and their interaction). Although screening for these conditions requires medical assessment, the social worker may be able to provide important contextual information about whether the confusional state has had a sudden onset, and whether there are factors in the person's life which may indicate susceptibility to confusion such as a high alcohol intake. Where confusion is more chronic and insidious, this may be related to serious physiological conditions such as advanced cancer, or organ failure, particularly of the kidneys or liver.

Activity 7.1 Discriminatory language and older people's mental health problems

Consider the following terms and identify any that would not be acceptable to use in any context, and specify the situations in which it would be appropriate to use the others:

- confused

- senile

- elderly mentally infirm

- living with dementia

- delirious.

Person-centred care

Possibly the most significant paradigm shift in recent years in working with people living with dementia has been the development of 'person-centred care'. Though this term can carry a generic meaning, within the context of dementia care it is identified almost exclusively with the work of the late Tom Kitwood (e.g., Kitwood and Benson 1995; Kitwood 1997). He and his colleagues are associated with the University of Bradford's Dementia Research Group formed in 1992, but later known as the Bradford Dementia Group. In his relatively short life Kitwood was ordained as an Anglican priest, became a schoolteacher in Uganda, later renounced his Christian beliefs, studied for a PhD in psychology and became a chartered psychologist and practising psychotherapist. The work that he undertook with colleagues in the 1990s assessing dementia services, developing assessment tools and developing principles of dementia care, was cut short by his sudden death in 1998 but he left behind a body of work that continues to evolve and influence service development.

The main principles of Kitwood and his Bradford colleagues' work derives from the humanistic psychology of Carl Rogers and his principle of unconditional regard for the individual. It has been commented that Kitwood's work is beset by ambiguity (Baldwin and Capstick 2007: xvii), apparent inconsistencies in some of the principles and approaches his work promotes, but undoubtedly his core message that services for people with dementia should start from the needs and perspectives of the individual, looking for the person behind the dementia, whilst simple, has had considerable impact.

Box 7.2   Kitwood's formula for explaining dementia

Kitwood conceptualised dementia in terms of an equation:

$$D = P + B + H + NI + SP$$

where D is dementia, P is the person's personality and personal resources, B stands for their biography, H their physical health, NI their neurological impairment and SP the social psychology of their environment. In proposing this formula Kitwood was rebalancing our approach to working with people living with dementia from a biologically based understanding of their impairment, to one that was multifactorial and gave equivalent weighting to the individual's life story and social environment. The situation within which the person is cared for can either support the expression of their individuality and enjoyment of social relationships or it can disempower and institutionalise them. Kitwood did not attribute the 'malignant social psychology' of the latter approach to the moral failings of individual workers, but saw this as sustained by the dominant 'culture of dementia care' that ignored the whole person in favour of treating a dehumanised 'patient' that only related to the symptoms of the disease.

An important aspect of the work of Bradford Dementia Group has been the development of tools for assessing whether care is producing beneficial outcomes for the individual, particularly in the light of the problems of verbal communication that are developed by many people living with dementia. Deriving from Kitwood and others' evaluation of day centre services, the Group has developed the Dementia Care Mapping approach. This is an assessment tool which contains indicators such as assertiveness, bodily relaxation, sensitivity to the needs of others, humour, creative self-expression, initiating social contact and expression of emotions. The scale derived from the Dementia Care Mapping approach can be used to evaluate the effectiveness of care environments and interventions (Brooker 2001).

Social interventions for dementia

In the last twenty years there has been a profusion of psychosocial interventions developed for use in the dementia field. It is understandable that in care settings these are sometimes adopted with enthusiasm because they hold out an optimistic orientation to working with people with dementia, but it is often difficult to assess objectively whether they are effective beyond these organisational considerations of providing a direction and framework for activity. The list of interventions includes reminiscence therapy, various forms of art therapies utilising music, dance, painting or sculpting, cognitive stimulation therapy (previously referred to as reality orientation therapy) and sensory stimulation. Systematic evaluations of the efficacy of these methods have been disappointing in their results, though this is not entirely surprising given the variations in the forms in which the therapies are delivered and the complexities of operationalising outcome measurements that can isolate whether change has taken place (Cheston and Bender 1999: 24). Where they are offered as genuine choices, and without punitive coercion to participate (which sometimes seemed to be a feature of reality orientation therapy), then there may be value in these therapies for their intrinsic opportunities for social interaction and validation, even if there is not a demonstrable relationship to an empirically demonstrated level of efficacy.

End of life care

At the present time the main forms of dementia are irreversible and those with the condition will eventually die from or with the condition, perhaps with a physical complication that may be associated with their increasing frailty. Despite this, and the numbers affected, there are few services designed specifically to provide palliative care for those living with dementia. Such a service might include advance care planning, symptom management (particularly pain, behavioural problems and depression), carer support and coordination of community support services. One model for doing this is to integrate the palliative approach into primary care services. One programme which evaluated such a service, delivered by specialist nurses attached to primary care teams, was able to demonstrate a high level of satisfaction with the quality of care, pain relief and control of the dying process (Shega et al., 2003). Increasingly, social workers are deployed within palliative care services (Payne and Reith 2009) and there seems to be a strong case for ensuring that they are involved in promoting the design and delivery of services for people with dementia. It is a recommendation of the NICE–SCIE national guidelines for dementia care practice that people with dementia who are dying should have the same access to palliative care services as those without dementia (National Collaborating Centre for Mental Health 2006b: 111).

Carers

Carers play a crucial role in relation to maintaining the autonomy and well-being of the person living with dementia. Not least, it is their resilience and coping capacity that is likely to be the determining factor in whether the person with dementia can remain living at home. At the same time, there is evidence that carers pay a high cost in terms of their own welfare and it has been suggested that this group carries a greater psychological and health burden than any other carer group (National Collaborating Centre for Mental Health 2006b: 280). Consequently, social workers need to give sufficient attention to identifying and supporting the needs of carers of individuals with dementia; a responsibility which is reinforced by statutory requirements under the Carers and Disabled Children's Act 2000 and the Carers (Equal Opportunities Act) 2004.

The role of the carer starts to become established at the earliest stages of the care pathway when assessment and diagnosis is taking place, though this is also the point at which their needs are often overlooked. This initial recognition by carers of the onset of dementia in a relative can initiate a period of anticipatory bereavement; a range of losses begin to be anticipated, whether it be the partner's loss of companionship, or a child's relinquishment of the relationship they have enjoyed with a parent. Whatever the type of relationship, entering into the role of carer is likely to curtail personal freedom, constrain the future plans of the carer and may precipitate insecurity of finances or employment, if the carer is still of working age. The caring responsibilities are also likely to involve new levels of personal intimacy and involvement in tasks of daily living. A renegotiation of the division of responsibilities in the household may be required as the carer takes on new areas of responsibility and skill, perhaps in managing aspects of the household finances or practical maintenance of the home. Research into caring indicates a range of responses including guilt and depression, and later onset of stress and exhaustion as the dementia develops and the responsibilities increase (Brodaty et al., 2003; Sorensen et al., 2002).

Information about services should be made available at the time of diagnosis. Professionals such as social workers may be desensitised to the limited levels of knowledge that people have about conditions such as dementia. A research study involving 205 carers found that most carers misattributed changes that were taking place in the behaviour of the person with dementia to causes other than the dementia, and over-estimated the person's responsibility for their cognitive and behavioural changes.

In addition a significant proportion of the carers believed the condition was reversible and the person with dementia would return to their previous level of functioning (Paton et al., 2004).

At the same time, the information provided to carers should be paced sensitively so that the carer does not become too demoralised. In the UK there is now fairly wide provision of information and support services, primarily provided by voluntary organisations, usually with local government funding, such as the Alzheimer's Society. There is a growing evidence-base in relation to what provides benefit for carers although there is a need for further research to identify the components of support that have most effectiveness. Sorensen et al.'s systematic review (2002) of carer interventions found that psychological therapy (notably CBT) and psychoeducation had the best results in relation to carers' rates of depression. Multi-component interventions, that is, those that combined a mix of interventions such as CBT, support groups, skills training and education had the best effect on measurements of carer burden and well-being. Attention should also be given to the development of programmes for carers that are attuned to gendered differences in approaches to caring, and the particular cultural needs of carers from black and ethnic minority groups (Adamson 2001).

Activity 7.2 Supporting carers to cope with difficult and challenging behaviour

SCIE has identified the following as some of the behaviours associated with the later stages of dementia that carers may find difficult or challenging. Consider how you would advise and support a carer to cope with each behaviour.

- Agitation. The person may become more agitated in the late afternoon and early evening. This is sometimes known as 'sundowning'.

- Aggression. The person may react aggressively if they feel threatened or cannot understand what is going on around them.

- Repetition. The person may rock backwards and forwards, use repetitive movements or keep calling out the same sound or word.

- Hallucinations. The person may see, smell, hear, taste or feel things that are not really there.

- Delusions. The person may develop distorted ideas about what is happening; these are often linked to hallucinations.

- Restlessness. Some people are restless and may wander around apparently aimlessly; this may be because they need more physical activity.

- Activity. The person may constantly wring their hands, pull at their clothes, tap, fidget or touch themselves inappropriately in public.

- Disinhibition. Some people become disinhibited, that is, they lose control of emotions or physical urges. A common example is overt sexualised behaviour.

- Inactivity. Periods of physical inactivity during which the person remains still, with their eyes open but not focused on anything, may increase.

(Adapted from Social Care Institute for Excellence 2007a)

Depression and old age

Because of the increasing priority attached to the development of dementia services, it is sometimes overlooked that the most prevalent mental health problem for older people is actually depression, with a prevalence rate that is equal to that for middle-age of 10 to 15 per cent (Social Care Institute for Excellence 2007b). The incidence and risks for older men are particularly high. Stereotypes of older age, which, as discussed above, are inherently negative, contribute to the invisibility of depression in older people. Thus, life course theories which portray old age as a period of disengagement or withdrawal support the interpretation of social withdrawal as 'normal'. This is compounded by the differing nature of help-seeking behaviour in older people. They are less likely to express suicidal thoughts, even though the rate of completed suicide is higher, particularly for men (Godfrey et al., 2005). Older people with depression are likely to visit their general practitioner more frequently, sometimes with multiple phys- ical problems that have no apparent explanation, leading to pejorative characterisations by doctors as 'frequent flyers'. Their mood may be agitated or anxious rather than depressed in the conventional sense. This mismatch between presentation and conventional diagnostic criteria for depression, means that even when it is recognised it is more likely to be categorised as 'mild' when in fact the person's level of distress is moderate or even severe.

As with depression in younger people, social factors play a significant role and may be one focus of intervention. Social isolation creates a state of vulnerability to depression. In older people there may well then be higher levels of triggering events which precipitate feelings of depression. These events can include loss such as bereavement of family and friends, deteriorating physical health, or worries about financial security. Relocation to live closer to well-meaning family who want their ageing parent to be more accessible can unintentionally compound depression through loss of a familiar environ- ment. Moving from independent living into residential care, often seen by the family as a 'solution', can exacerbate the risk of depression.

The range of social, psychological and physical treatments that are evidence-based as effective for younger people are equally so for older people. They are often under-used by practitioners because of the 'normalisation' of depression in older people. Reducing social isolation is obviously an important consideration and domiciliary and community-based services can be helpful in this respect. Risks also have to be considered as suicide rates are higher in older people, particularly men; overall morbidity rates for depressed older people are twice those for non-depressed individuals (Godfrey et al., 2005). As for younger people, the earlier intervention can be offered, the better the likelihood of improvement in the person's mental state.

A final consideration in relation to depression in older people is that it is often associated with dementia. This may be the product of despair and pessimism related to the receipt of a diagnosis of dementia, environmental loss factors such as those discussed above, or the quality of the caring environment. The advice of NICE–SCIE guidelines for dementia care is that assessment for co-existing depression should begin with these environmental factors (National Collaboration Centre for Mental Health 2006b: 230). Research evidence reviewed in the preparation of these guidelines (Gould and Kendall 2007 describes the methodology) indicates that people with dementia and depression value meeting in groups for mutual support and social activities. There is also some emerging evidence that cognitive behavioural therapy for individuals can be helpful. People with depression and dementia have also expressed appreciation of feeling helped by a range of psychosocial forms of intervention such as multi-sensory stimulation (so-called snoezelen rooms), relaxation training and pet-assisted therapy.

Longstanding mental health problems in old age

There is a tendency, and it probably again reflects a stereotypical view of old age carried by professionals, to think of mental health problems in older age as only related to dementia and depression. It should be appreciated that some people who have not experienced a major mental disorder during their working-age adulthood may develop significant problems in older age. A significant proportion of psychiatric hospital admissions in older people are for mania (Shulman 1993). Sometimes this is precipitated by an acute physical illness. Many such individuals have a history of depression though in a manic phase they often present as irritable, labile or perplexed. The prognosis is generally good, provided that – as with mania in younger people – treatment is timely. For the social worker, intervention is likely to be as for younger people with a bipolar disorder, providing encouragement to engage with treatment, supporting carers and helping manage the consequences of reckless behaviour.

Ten per cent of people who develop schizophrenia do so after the age of 60 (Godfrey et al., 2005). Whether this should be regarded as very late-onset schizophrenia, or whether this is a distinct condition remains contested within psychiatry. Sometimes this may be manifested in the form of circumscribed persecutory delusions in the context of otherwise normal social and psychological functioning: perhaps the idea that a relative or friend is plotting against the individual. Social workers and domiciliary support workers will often experience seeking to support people whose florid complaints about conspiracies of relatives or neighbours against the individual will be causing severe stress to their personal relationships, whilst still managing to live independently in the community. Other individuals may present with delusions or hallucinations that correspond to acute schizophrenia with first rank symptoms. It has been noted that the onset of these problems often follows periods of long-term social isolation. Of course, it may be difficult to disentangle the direction of the causal relationship, as isolation may be a behavioural response to insidious development of delusional thinking. Nevertheless, people with these difficulties can make a good recovery, albeit their insight into their problems may remain limited. Older people with delusions should be considered for the same range of interventions as younger people, although medical practitioners are likely to be wary of possible side effects, particularly elevated risks of vascular complications with some atypical antipsychotic drugs.

What is commonly overlooked is that adults who have intermittently or enduringly experienced other mental health problems throughout their lives will live into older age and retain their needs for services and support. This has always been the case but, with increased longevity in the population, a greater number of people with problems that began in earlier adulthood will live beyond the age at which old age is normally defined. Estimating and projecting the numbers involved are difficult because many are probably lost from services and are 'hidden' and estimates vary from 11 to 60 per 100,000 (Jolley et al., 2002; Jolley et al., 2004). These individuals are sometimes referred to in the psychiatric literature as 'graduates', because they graduate from being the responsibility of adult services to older age services though this term is rather discriminatory because of its flippancy and implication of a burden on services. The most common form of mental disorder that older people with enduring mental health problems present is schizophrenia, though some people persist with experiencing bipolar affective disorder late into their lives (Jolley et al., 2004). It has been an enduring myth of mental health workers that these conditions 'burn out' in middle age, but this is sometimes not the case and results in services not being offered. Such individuals have a number of threats to their well-being. They may become a victim of service demarcation if there are not flexible arrangements either for the transfer of care from adult to old-age services, including loss of continuity of established relationships with practitioners, but they may also not have expert help to deal with the complex interaction of physical and mental health problems associated with older age; for instance, that they may experience co-morbidities of an enduring psychotic condition and dementia.

Key points

- Despite negative stereotypes of the ageing process, most people retain their mental capabilities and contribute positively to society. However, as people live longer so the number of individuals living with age-related mental health problems such as dementia will grow.

- 'Dementia' is an umbrella term for a range of progressive, terminal brain diseases which lead to memory impairment and other psychological and behavioural problems. The most common forms of dementia in older age are Alzheimer's disease, vascular dementia, and Lewy bodies dementia.

- Psychosocial approaches to dementia, such as Kitwood's or Cheston and Benders', focus on the uniqueness of the individual and the changes that ensue in their social roles and communication.

Kitwood's approach is rooted in Carl Rogers' principle of unconditional regard for the individual and has been a transformational influence in dementia care.

- End of life, or palliative, care is an important dimension of dementia care but has received insufficient attention within mainstream services.

- Carers play a crucial role in maintaining the autonomy and well-being of the person living with dementia, but often they pay a high price in terms of their own mental health. Their own needs should be assessed and responded to by social workers.

- Although dementia is the main focus of concern regarding mental health in old age, the most prevalent form of mental health problem for older people is depression, and this is particularly found in residential and day care.

- Services for older people also tend to overlook the needs of people who developed a problem such as schizophrenia or bipolar disorder during their working-age life, and who continue to experience recurrences of these disorders.

Key reading

Cantley, C. (ed.) (2001) *A Handbook of Dementia Care*, Buckingham: Open University Press.

National Collaborating Centre for Mental Health (2006) *A NICE-SCIE Guideline on Supporting People with Dementia and their Carers in Health and Social Care, National Clinical Practice Guideline Number 42*, London: The British Psychological Society and Gaskell.

Tanner, D. and Harris, J. (2008) *Working with Older People*, London: Routledge.

8 Risk and dangerousness

By the end of this chapter you should have an understanding of:

- Sociological interest in changing perceptions of risk and their influence on the development of mental health policy

- Risk factors in relation to suicide

- The role that mental health problems sometimes, albeit rarely, play in relation to risk to others

- Guidance for social workers in relation to the identification and management of risk and dangerousness

- The situations in which compulsory treatment is possibly to be considered as an option and the powers available under the 1983 and 2007 Mental Health Acts

- The social work role in relation to compulsion including acting as an Approved Mental Health Practitioner

- The contribution of the social perspective to decision-making in Mental Health Review Tribunals

- The range of services for mentally disordered offenders

- Practising as a social worker in secure mental health settings.

The nature of risk

The concept of the 'risk society' has been prominent in sociology for over a decade (e.g., Beck 1992; Giddens 1991). Broadly, the risk society perspective encapsulates two observations. The first is the apparent paradox that the more technologically developed society becomes and able to manage and remedy adversities, the more society seems convinced that the world is a dangerous and threatening place. The second is the apparent collapse of deference towards experts, with the consequent effect of neutralising their efforts to persuade people that the world is not as dangerous as they think. There are a number of examples to support this hypothesis from subjective fears of experience such as flying in aeroplanes to the perception of parents that their children are at ubiquitous risk of abduction and harm from strangers. These attitudes and the behaviours we adopt in response to them may themselves have unintended negative outcomes: children fail to learn skills of managing everyday challenges because they are over-protected by parents; parents place their children at risk of impairment or even death because they cannot be reassured that a triple vaccine for measles, mumps and rubella does not place their child at risk of autism (Baron-Cohen 2009). Webb (2006) has analysed in some depth the effects that the 'risk society' has had on social work including the preoccupation with risk management and defensive approaches to practice.

The attitudes and behaviours that Beck, Giddens and others have identified as characterising the risk society have relevance for policy and practice in relation to people with mental health problems. Isolated instances of failures in individual cases leading to harmful behaviours by people who have been in contact with mental health services become exaggerated to generate perceptions that such people are inherently dangerous and need to be controlled and even confined. One explanation for this is the low level of statistical comprehension amongst the general population, such that individuals cannot interpret simple descriptive statistics and understand the probabilities of risk that derive from them (Gigerenzer 2002). In addition, at a societal level, there are processes of 'amplification of deviancy', as described by the sociologist Stanley Cohen (1987), whereby, given the right public climate, single or a few instances of a problem become magnified by the media, politicians and pundits into a 'moral panic' and fears of imminent collapse of public safety.

Within British public policy these issues have been played out at a relatively prominent level in recent years. A case study of this could be the debates leading to the introduction of Community Treatment Orders (CTOs), permitting drug treatments to be taken under compulsion by individuals living in the community, eventually legislated for in the 2007 Mental Health Act. Various commentators argued that this amendment to the 1983 Mental Health Act was provoked primarily by selective media attention to isolated homicides and serious assaults by users of mental health services that became the ammunition for populist newspapers claiming the failure of deinstitutionalisation and care in the community (Taylor and Gunn 1999). In turn the cause of compulsory treatment became a touchstone for politicians anxious to avoid being seen as lenient on matters of law and order. The government has pressed ahead with the introduction of CTOs despite its own review of the research evidence for their efficacy in six countries where they are currently used showing little evidence of positive effects (Churchill 2007).

A more subtle impact of a policy that imposes social control on people with a mental health problem has been the progressive extension of public order legislation that, intentionally or otherwise, incorporates and criminalises people whose underlying problem may be related to their mental health. For example, Anti Social Behaviour orders (ASBOs), created by the Crime and Disorder Act 1998, ostensibly are intended to constrain nuisance behaviour in public places. Their use by courts, which are often not minded to ask for expert assessments of a defendant's mental health state, often leads to people with mental health problems being placed on an order. Such orders are civil, but a breach of the conditions of the order – often by someone who does not have the mental capacity to comply – will result in the issue being dealt with as a criminal matter. The Sainsbury Centre for Mental Health claims that around one-third of ASBOs are made in relation to people who have a mental health problem (Sainsbury Centre for Mental Health 2007).

In the main people with mental health problems are managed under the powers of the Mental Health Acts. Campbell and Heginbotham (1991) have argued that mental health legislation is inherently discriminatory. They contend that dangerousness should be considered as a quality that is acted out by a cross-section of people in society and not restricted to people with a mental disorder. To legislate for the constraint of people with a mental disorder who are potentially dangerous as a special category, they argue, is to discriminate against those people. Their proposal is that if society wishes to pass laws that are designed to prevent individuals behaving dangerously, then they should be generic, applicable to the whole population, and not limited to mental health patients. Their argument provokes objections about whether in reality it is progressive to have such a radical extension of indeterminate sentencing, but it does focus attention on the justifiability of differentially constraining the liberties of people by virtue of them being diagnosed with a mental health problem.

This chapter addresses various practice-related aspects of risk and dangerousness in relation to mental disorder, but seeks to do so in cognisance of this sociologically informed awareness that these are topics that are highly problematic. So, we consider them as topics that are socially produced by the anxieties of our times whilst at the same time are realistic in that social workers do have pragmatic needs to acknowledge and respond to those rare events in mental health practice where the safety the public or the individual with a mental health problem is implicated. It is evident from even a cursory awareness of the statistics that people with a mental health problems are at far greater risk of harming themselves than anyone else. People with mental health problems also find themselves placed at greater risk of harm by virtue of being treated within the mental health system, not least the high levels of assault on service users in acute services (Mental Health Act Commission 2008). Nevertheless, at the same time there are situations and psychological states that practitioners may encounter that do place the general public at greater levels of risk.

Risk, dangerousness and mental disorder

Risk to self: suicide

As we have seen, by far the greatest danger to the person with a mental disorder is from self-harm and suicide. Conditions such as depression and schizophrenia carry with them risks of suicide that are considerably higher than the average for the general population (Harris and Barraclough 1997; Appleby et al., 1999). In terms of demographics, suicide rates are influenced by a range of social factors such as age, gender and ethnicity. Events in someone's earlier life can also predispose individuals towards suicide. Research by the author found that amongst men who had been sexually abused in childhood rates of suicidal thinking were ten times greater than in the general population (O'Leary and Gould 2008). Most individuals who have experienced early trauma have mechanisms for dealing with the effects in later life, but for a significant proportion there are continuing problems in living. Understanding the psychological mechanisms that influence adaptation to abuse and having the interviewing skills to elicit earlier experiences of trauma are important parts of the mental health social worker's repertoire. However, once again we should be wary of the 'ecological fallacy'. When social workers are assessing an individual's level of risk of attempting suicide, they should be alert to the possibility that a service user falls within a higher risk category – for example, an unemployed, older man, or young Asian woman (Raleigh and Balarajan 1992) – but it is always possible that an individual does not fall into such a category and yet may seriously be contemplating suicide. Each assessment should consider the unique features of the person's history and social circumstances.

When a person is seriously depressed, their level of motivation may be so low that even the initiative needed to take their own life may be lacking. It may seem paradoxical that the risks of suicide rise as the mental health of the severely depressed person improves and their mood lifts; this may be the point at which they regain the level of self-motivation that is necessary to manage the practicalities of killing themselves. Another factor relevant to situations where 'watchful waiting' and monitoring are required is the time delay in anti-depressant medication starting to take effect. SSRIs and other drug treatments for depression are likely to take several days to a few weeks to begin to affect the person's mood. It could be a tragic mistake to assume that once someone has accepted medication that the risk of suicide is ended at that point.

Many lay people, and even some professionals, hesitate in interviewing someone who may be suicidal in directly asking that person whether they intend to take their own life. The consensus in the literature is that the intention to commit suicide is never triggered by making reference to this. Practitioners need to have the confidence to ask direct questions. Providing the opportunity for the service user to offload their feelings about ending their life and could in itself be cathartic. In response, the practitioner may then need to be proactive in taking steps to make the situation safe, perhaps removing the means by which the person intended to take their life, such as a stockpile of medication, or to arrange an assessment with a view to admission to hospital. It should be remembered that the occupational groups with the highest suicide rates tend to be those with easiest access to means of taking their own lives, such as doctors and dentists with access to drugs, and farmers with firearms (Department of Health 1999).

Finally, we should not confine our reflections on suicide to depression. People living with psychotic conditions such as schizophrenia also have very high risks of suicide (Brown 1997). We can only speculate, but it seems likely that some people find the hallucinatory voices they hear, or their delusional beliefs, so terrifying or oppressive that ultimately they find life too difficult to carry on. The experience of psychosis can also lead to social isolation so that when crises are reached, the person does not have supportive networks at hand. These are all factors that need to be considered in relation to care planning in working with people with schizophrenia or other psychotic conditions.

Risk to others

Although overall, people with mental health problems are no more likely than those without a mental health problem to behave dangerously, there are characteristics and situational factors that contribute to elevated levels of risk to others (Prins 1999). In making an assessment of developing a care plan these need to be considered and their effects anticipated. Research to develop precise actuarial methods for predicting dangerousness may be fraught with difficulty, but these factors should not be ignored, rather they need to be considered and weighted using reflective professional judgement:

- *Mental disorder in combination with substance misuse.* The effects in all of us of alcohol and narcotics are generally to disinhibit behaviour and weaken the internalised controls that usually operate; people's behaviour under the influence of these substances tends to be more aggressive or socially inappropriate. In individuals with a mental health problem the effect may be to further distort the norms and insight that would otherwise guide their behaviour, sometimes leading to chaotic or even violent behaviour. For example, someone who holds delusional beliefs that another person is spying on them, may be more likely to take retaliatory action against that person when they are inebriated. A detailed clinical and social history may well reveal patterns of behaviour where consumption of alcohol or illegal drugs when someone is acutely unwell triggers antisocial behaviour. One intervention for work with such a person may be to help them to recognise and manage the consequences of substance misuse when unwell.

- *Passivity experiences and command hallucinations.* We have seen that one form of delusional belief in schizophrenia and other related conditions can be that a person believes they are being controlled by external forces that direct their actions. Acting on such beliefs, a person may consider that normal moral constraints on their behaviour may be suspended or irrelevant. Peter Sutcliffe, the so-called Yorkshire Ripper, believed that God was instructing him to rid the world of prostitutes. This is thankfully a very extreme example (and he was not known at the time of his offences to psychiatric services) but it makes the point that practitioners need to pay attention to the content of hallucinations and delusions, and they should be responded to seriously if there are implications that, if acted on, others will be put at risk.

- *Paranoid delusions.* Another form of psychotic experience that we have considered is the irrational but persistent belief that a person is being persecuted or placed in danger. Because this false belief is held by the person experiencing it to be absolutely true, their response may be to defend themselves by attacking their perceived persecutor. As with command hallucinations, the intention to act upon these mistaken beliefs should be responded to by the practitioner to protect those potentially at risk. The social worker has to be additionally alert to the possibility that they may become incorporated into these delusional beliefs and so themselves become placed at risk.

- *Lack of empathy for the pain of others.* Under certain mental conditions some individuals seem to lose (or have never developed) the capacity to identify with the pain or distress that others feel. In some personality disorders this may be an inherent part of the person's personality, such as in antisocial personality disorder where individuals may be oblivious to the hurt that they inflict on others. In psychotic states, the delusional beliefs held by someone, as we have discussed in relation to paranoia and passivity experiences, may seem to diminish an individual's capacity for empathy. Sometimes this tendency is revealed in a person's preoccupation with sadistic or violent fantasy materials, such as sadomasochistic pornography or literature. This can be a significant element in compiling a forensic assessment.

- *Depressive mood and feelings of nihilism.* There have been a number of high-profile cases where an individual becomes so depressed and pessimistic about their circumstances that they feel the only solution for themselves and those they love is to kill their family and commit suicide ('familicide') (Gould 2001). In some cases the situation is precipitated by a relationship breakdown and problems of child custody or access. Sometimes they are not predicted because the perpetrator (usually a male) is able to disguise the extent of their depression and the eventual carnage seems to have come 'out of the blue'. Nevertheless, sometimes individuals give indications that their loved ones are 'too good for this terrible world' which are not recognised as portents of disaster. Mental health social workers and child protection social workers should consider risk factors for familicide in working with families where a parent or carer seems suicidally depressed.

Working in situations where there are levels of risk such as these to be assessed and monitored is not for every social worker. This needs to be confronted honestly as practitioners with persistently high levels of anxiety, or who are inhibited from acting authoritatively when necessary, are less likely to be able to function effectively to protect themselves or others. It requires high levels of self-knowledge in order to monitor one's own response to situations of risk and to take action. Not least it requires attention to processes that in days more influenced by psychoanalytic theory were referred to as 'transference' and 'counter transference'. This means being able to tune in to one's own feelings about a situation, to disentangle rational from irrational feelings about interactions with service users, and to have a developed sense of intuition about situations that are going wrong. This kind of forensic work also requires good supervision and responsive support structures within organisations to protect practitioners from burn-out. In 2007 the Department of Health issued a guidance document called *Best Practice in Managing Risk: principles and guidance for best practice in the assessment and management of risk to self and others in mental health services* which emphasises the need for open, non-defensive team cultures:

> Risk management plans should be developed by multidisciplinary and multiagency teams operating in an open, democratic and transparent culture that embraces reflective practice.
>
> (Department of Health 2007d: 6)

Activity 8.1 Assessing risk

David is a 35-year-old man who is described in records as white British. He is unemployed and lives alone in a bedsitter in an inner-city area that is ethnically diverse, characterised by high levels of multi-occupied housing and social deprivation. David is well known to mental health services, and has had several admissions to hospital for treatment, some of them under sections 2 and 3 of the Mental Health Act 1983, though he has never been a risk to others, but he has disengaged from services for more than six months. His diagnosis has always been uncertain, with some disagreement between psychiatrists who have treated him in the past as to whether David has schizophrenia or bipolar disorder. A constant feature in his history of mental health problems has been that when his level of psychotic thinking is rising he tends to smoke increasing amounts of cannabis as a means of containing his level of distress.

You are a social worker who in the past has been David's care manager and who has been asked to visit David because his father has phoned the Community Mental Health Team to say that David is becoming increasingly hostile, is wearing a sheath knife on his belt, his self-care is deteriorating and he is continuously smoking cannabis. The father is particularly upset because David is saying that his real father is Adolf Hitler and that he has 'a duty to continue his work'; these are pre-occupations that David has never presented before.

What would be your considerations in deciding how and when a visit to David should be made? What would you consider to be salient risk factors for David and others that could be present in this situation?

The use of compulsion in mental health practice

The use of compulsion in mental health practice is sometimes controversial and for some social workers reluctance to participate in depriving people with mental health problems of their liberty is a reason why they work in other specialisms, or outside the statutory sector. Historically, there seems to be a pendulum that swings between prioritising the role of the legal system in depriving mentally disordered people of their liberties, and legislating to give psychiatrists predominant jurisdiction on the apparent basis that 'doctor knows best'. Social workers in their various guises as Mental Welfare Officer (the 1959 Mental Health Act), Approved Social Workers (1983 Mental Health Act) and Approved Mental Health Professionals (2007 Mental Health Act) to varying degrees hold the ring as the independent referees of these two tendencies.

Intriguingly, the swing of the pendulum seems to take approximately twenty-five years for legislative action and reaction to occur in relation to mental health, with the major reforming Acts falling in 1933, 1959, 1983 and 2007. The 1959 Mental Health Act marked a swing of the pendulum towards medical discretion through the enhancement of the powers of the Responsible Medical Officer (RMO). The 1983 Mental Health Act subsequently reasserted some of the authority of legal process with the strengthening of means for legal recourse for patients; for instance, through enhanced access to the Mental Health Review Tribunal, supported by European case law which asserted the rights of patients to judicial review of their detention, and the eventual incorporation of European human rights legislation into British law. It is arguable that the recent amendments to the 1983 Act that are contained in the 2007 Mental Health Act in some respects swing back towards medical discretion through a broader definition of mental disorder, and the introduction of compulsory treatment in the community.

Undoubtedly a challenge for reformers of mental health legislation has been the changing role of the hospital in the management of people with severe mental health problems. The presumption of past mental health law, including the 1983 Mental Health Act, was that care and treatment were typically delivered in the context of admission to hospital for inpatient treatment. This became increasingly questionable with the process of de-institutionalisation. The need to modernise mental health law to address the reality of community-based care as the dominant paradigm, and the increasing moral panic about mental illness and dangerousness, have been persistent drivers in political discourse about the use of compulsory powers. It was the underlying principle of the 1983 Mental Health Act that treatment should be delivered in the 'least restrictive environment'. This phrase was never directly incorporated into the legislation but the authorities detaining a person with a mental health disorder have to be of the view that detention in hospital is the most appropriate way of providing for the patient's mental health needs (1983 Mental Health Act s.13(2)).

Now, after much debate, the 2007 Mental Health Act creates powers to require people to accept treatment in the community under the Community Treatment Order. A remarkable effect of the legislation as it slowly passed through parliament was that it galvanised most of the mental health community into opposition to it, with many unlikely bedfellows such as the Royal College of Psychiatry, the major mental health voluntary organisations, and service user led groups working in alliance (see the Mental Health Alliance website at www.mentalhealthalliance.org.uk). Eventually a modified version of the legislation was enacted and has been implemented from November 2008. Confusingly, the 2007 Mental Health Act does not replace the 1983 Mental Health Act, it amends it, so we now have to understand the composite effect of these two pieces of legislation. It is beyond the scope of this book to explain comprehensively this complex legislation (and social workers will now also need to be familiar with legislation relating to the mental capacity of service users, namely the Mental Capacity Act 2005 and the amendments introduced by the deprivation of liberty safeguards). Social workers working in this area are strongly recommended to consult specialist manuals, most notably the eleventh edition of Richard Jones's authoritative Mental Health Act Manual (Jones 2008), the author being qualified as both a solicitor and a social worker! The basic scope of the Mental Health Acts is explained in Box 8.1.

Box 8.1   Scope of the Mental Health Act 1983 and Mental Health Act 2007

The 1983 Mental Health Act as amended by the 2007 Act applies to those deemed to be suffering from a mental disorder (Section 1). This Act replaces the four categories of mental disorder previously given in the Section 1 of the 1983 Mental Health Act – mental illness, mental impairment, severe mental impairment and psychopathic disorder. The stated intention of the government in making this change was to provide, 'a simpler single definition of mental disorder . . . this simple single definition will also make the Act easier for clinicians use and for other to understand' (*Hansard*, HL Vol. 687, col. 657). The concern of many is that the new definition is so broad and subject to the discretion of clinicians that it could widen the net of compulsion by medicalising those persons whose problems are social or whose behaviour is considered deviant. The Act excludes those whose primary problem is dependence on drugs or alcohol, but these are the only stated exclusions. Although *ICD-10* and *DSM-IV* do not include diagnoses based on sexual preferences, strictly interpreted there is nothing in the Act to prevent clinicians applying diagnostic criteria that are not in the manuals. The counter-argument is that the definition of mental disorder needs to be open-ended to allow for the evolution of medical understanding of psychiatric illnesses, but no doubt there will be legal challenges to establish the limits of this extended scope of the legislation.

Having established that a person has a mental disorder within the meaning of the Act, compulsory detention requires that at least one of three criteria is satisfied. It is a common misconception amongst social workers that at least two criteria have to be satisfied, but the criteria are linked by the word *or* rather than *and*:

3(2) An application for admission for treatment may be made in respect of a patient on the grounds that –

a)   He is suffering from [mental disorder] of a nature or degree which makes it appropriate for him to receive medical treatment in a hospital; and

b)   [. . . .]

> c) It is necessary for the health or safety of the patient or for the protection of other persons that he should receive such treatment and it cannot be provided unless he is detained under this section.

The error sometimes made by mental health practitioners is to presume that safety of the patient or protection of others has to be present as a risk factor to justify detention, but as the wording of the Act clearly shows, an order for detention in hospital can be made purely on the grounds of the health of the individual, another insertion of medical discretion (some would say paternalism) into the legislation. It has also been established that 'health' in this context refers to mental as well as physical health (Mental Health Act Commission *Second Biennial Report, 1985*–87 para 1.3). These criteria pertain not only to detention for treatment (section 3 of the 1983 Mental Health Act), but also for detention for assessment (section 2). 'Safety' includes act of self-harm including suicide, but also includes the possibility of harm from others if his or her behaviour while mentally disordered renders them likely to be provocative to others with subsequent risk of attack. 'Protection of other persons' includes psychological as well as physical harm to others (Code of Practice para 4.8). Thus, emotional harm to a carer could come within the meaning of this criterion (Jones 2008: 30), and that might mean that damage to property could be a factor if it, for example, means damage to the belongings or dwelling of a carer causes psychological harm.

The social work role in compulsion

From Mental Welfare Officer to Approved Mental Health Professional

In the United Kingdom the role of social workers in exercising statutory powers under mental health legislation has been distinct within the profession. The 1959 Mental Health Act created Mental Welfare Officers (MWOs): social workers who were mandated to make applications for compulsory admissions to mental hospitals (so-called 'sectioning') in conjunction with medical practitioners whose recommendations for admission could only be effected with the agreement of the MWO. Despite the moral panic around child protection in the 1970s ensuing from the Maria Colwell case, it was in mental health that social workers were first mandated to take post-qualifying training. The 1983 Mental Health Act redesignated MWOs as Approved Social Workers (ASWs) who, like MWOs before them, had the responsibility of making applications where compulsory admission to mental hospital was necessary.

Despite considerable opposition from the British Association of Social Workers (British Association of Social Workers 2006), the 2007 Mental Health Act has redefined the role only previously available to social workers and redesignated Approved Social Workers as Approved Mental Health Professionals (AMHPs), making the role available to clinical professionals such as psychologists, nurses or occupational therapists. It was argued by the policy-makers that the continuing extension of statutory mental health duties, combined with the ageing profile of the ASW workforce and problems of recruitment and retention of social work staff, meant that in order to avoid future shortfalls of personnel available to undertake tasks such as applications for compulsory admissions the pool of potential recruits would have to be widened to include other professionals.

The counter-argument of the British Association of Social Workers has been that this would seriously dilute the social perspective within statutory mental health procedures, which derived from the insights of professionals who have a social science-based education and whose value-base draws significantly from anti-discriminatory and anti-oppressive perspectives. Also, the discharge of statutory duties by professionals who were employees of the National Health Service, used to working within the hierarchical relationships of clinical teams, and whose educational background lent more towards the medical model, would not have the independence previously enjoyed by the Approved Social Worker.

Various compromises have been enacted within the final version of the 2007 Mental Health Act to assuage the critics of the AMHP proposals. The first is that it remains the responsibility of the local authority to train and authorise practitioners to act as AMHPs, thus preserving the relationship with councils with social services responsibilities, and giving them some independence from health authorities (though it must be questionable how real that independence is when an individual's main contract of employment remains with the NHS). Furthermore, the responsibility for developing the curriculum for training AMHPs remain with the General Social Care Council, the education and registration body for social work, so maintaining a professional and institutional connection to social work. Henceforth, when we discuss 'the social work role' in relation to statutory duties of the AMHP, these considerations also apply to other professionals who might be undertaking that role, such as occupational therapists, nurses and psychologists.

Despite being approved by the local authority as competent to act under mental health law, the AMHP remains, as did the ASW, individually liable for their own practice. This has always been an additional pressure for social workers acting in this role, as they are aware that they could find themselves sued for any lapse in their practice though in reality these legal actions are few and far between.

Compulsory admission to hospital

When a local social services authority has reason to believe that an application for admission to hospital (or a guardian application – see below) may be necessary, then arrangements must be made for an AMHP to consider the patient's case on their behalf (section 13, 1983 Mental Health Act). If the AMHP is satisfied that an admission ought to be made, then they have a duty to do so (section 13 (a)). The AMHP has to take into account the wishes of the relative of the patient, the wishes expressed by the patient and 'any other relevant circumstances'. A crucial requirement that has existed since the passing of the 1983 Mental Health Act has been that the patient should be interviewed, 'in a suitable manner'. This requirement was inserted for two reasons: the first, a concern that some social workers might be prepared to 'rubber stamp' an application under pressure from psychiatrists or family without a proper assessment of the circumstances; the second, a concern that individuals with hearing impairments were at risk of being sectioned if an appropriate interpreter was not provided. This concern became broadened in the Code of Practice to become a requirement that the wider communication needs of the patient should be considered, that a face-to-face interview should take place and that issues of language and culture should be taken into account in ensuring that a full and sensitive assessment takes place. This requirement remains an important statutory basis for social workers acting as AMHPs to ensure that assessments under the Mental Health Acts are based on anti-discriminatory principles. This is crucial given the continuing over-representation of black and minority ethnic patients in the detained hospital population (Commission for Healthcare Audit and Inspection 2007).

The nearest relative of a patient has a right (1983 Mental Health Act Section 13 (4)) to require a local social services authority to direct an AMHP to assess a patient's need for admission. Reasonable care needs to be taken in interpreting what constitutes a 'request', and judgement has to be exercised in deciding whether a phrase such as 'something has to be done about him' constitutes a request under this section of the Act. Where an assessment is subsequently made and the AMHP decides that an application for admission is not justified, the reasons for this decision have to be relayed to the nearest relative in writing.

Sometimes gaining access to someone to interview them in a suitable manner is not straightforward; it may be unclear whether someone is residing at an address but unwilling to speak to mental health professionals, or they are in residence but actively refusing to cooperate with the process of assessment. In situations of urgency where there is concern about the safety of the person or others, the AMHP may seek a warrant from a magistrate so that police can effect entry to the property and take the patient to a place of safety for assessment. Once again, these are situations that cause social workers deep concern about civil liberties. Indeed, there is a risk of contravention of article 8 of the European Convention on Human Rights, constituting a threat to the private life of the individual, and the action of the AMHP must be proportional (Jones 2008: 505). These anxieties have to be balanced against concerns that sometimes there may be a direct threat to the life of the service user (for example if they are suicidal) or others.

Guardianship

Sometimes the least restrictive alternative might be that a person is placed under a guardianship order rather than admitted to hospital (1983 Mental Health Act section 7). This requires a person to receive visits from an appointed guardian, to reside at a place directed by the guardian and to attend as required by the guardian for treatment. Local social service authorities are under a duty to receive applications for guardianship and to appoint a guardian, which could be an AMHP but can be anyone in a position to take responsibility for the patient's welfare. The antecedents for guardianship were statutory powers for supervision in the community of people with learning difficulties who struggled with the practical management of their affairs. The hope under the 1983 Act was that guardianship would be a means of maintaining patients in the community without compulsory admission to hospital, an antecedent to community supervised treatment. The use of guardianship orders has been very patchy, reflecting local variations in policies. In some areas it has been tried, particularly in relation to people with dementia living in residential care, as a means of clarifying the legal powers of care staff. In many situations its usefulness is limited: a person willing to comply with guardianship probably has the capacity not to need the order to be in place; where a person resists the directions of their guardian, the only sanction is to consider a compulsory admission to hospital, a course of action which is available without the order.

Activity 8.2 Social perspectives and the approved mental health professional

Read the sections in this chapter on the role of the Approved Mental Health Professional and any other sources you can identify in relation to the social work role in relation to the use of compulsion under the Mental Health Acts 2007 and 1983. What part can social workers play in ensuring that social perspectives are considered in decision-making processes that take place under the auspices of the Mental Health Acts? What might be the implications for social perspectives of the authorisation of clinical professionals such as nurses or psychologists as Approved Mental Health Professionals?

Social workers and Mental Health Review Tribunals

Patients who are detained in hospital for assessment or treatment are discharged under supervision in the community, subject to CTOs or who are subject to a guardianship, all have recourse to a Mental Health Review Tribunal (MHRT). This is a judicial body that is part of the health, education and social care chamber of the Tribunal Judiciary and completely independent of the detaining health authority, though it meets wherever the patient is detained. An MHRT comprises a legally qualified chairperson (referred to as the tribunal judge), a medical member and a lay member who has knowledge of mental health services (often individuals from social work backgrounds). The patient has a right to legal representation, which is funded by legal aid, and the tribunal conducts its deliberations by means of cross-examination of the key individuals responsible for the care and detention of the patient. The responsibility is on the detaining authority to prove its case that detention under the Mental Health Acts is warranted, not for the patient to prove that they do not require compulsory detention or supervision. Reports have to be placed before the tribunal, including a report on the social circumstances of the patient, and the MHRT will cross-examine the author of that report or their representative. The social report does not have to be presented by a social worker, but in most instances they are, and this is an important opportunity for the social perspectives relevant to a patient's welfare to be considered. A competent social report should provide a comprehensive assessment of the patient's circumstances; aspects which should be covered are listed in Box 8.2.

> **Box 8.2 Matters to be addressed in the social circumstances report for a Mental Health Review Tribunal**
>
> The social circumstances report must include the following information:
>
> a) the patient's home and family circumstances;
>
> b) in so far as it is practicable, and except in restricted cases, a summary of the views of the patient's nearest relative, unless (having consulted the patient) the person compiling the report thinks it would be inappropriate to consult the nearest relative;
>
> c) in so far as it is practicable, the views of any person who plays a substantial part in the care of the patient but is not professionally concerned with it;
>
> d) the views of the patient, including his concerns, hopes and beliefs in relation to the Tribunal proceedings and their outcome;
>
> e) the opportunities for employment and the housing facilities available to the patient;
>
> f) what (if any) community support is or will be made available to the patient and its effectiveness, if the patient is discharged from hospital;
>
> g) the patient's financial circumstances (including his entitlement to benefits);
>
> h) an assessment of the patient's strengths and any other positive factors that the Tribunal should be aware of in coming to a view on whether he should be discharged;
>
> i) an assessment of the extent to which the patient or other persons would be likely to be at risk if the patient is discharged by the Tribunal, and how any such risks could best be managed.
>
> (From Practice Direction, Health, Education and Social Care Chamber: Mental Health Cases 2009)

Services for mentally disordered offenders

A relatively small number of mental health social workers choose to practise in secure settings, with people who present acute management problems to mainstream services because of their challenging behaviour, or who are detained because they have committed criminal offences and have a mental disorder. This latter area of work is sometimes referred to as forensic psychiatry, a term which covers the assessment, treatment and rehabilitation of mentally disordered offenders. It is well known that many people with mental health problems are inappropriately dealt with through the criminal justice system and imprisonment; it has been estimated that 70 per cent of prisoners have two or more mental disorders (Crook 2007). Increasingly priority has been placed on attempting to identify those who would be more appropriately managed by health and social care services and by diverting them accordingly. There are a number of points in the pathway of someone with a mental health problem who has committed an offence at which their needs might be identified. Many magistrates' courts and police stations now have mental health assessment schemes available to them, the purpose of which is to consider whether an individual can be appropriately diverted from the criminal justice system. Interventions are made on the basis that early access to health and social care will help prevent further deterioration in a person's condition, reduce the likelihood of re-offending and avoid unsuitable use of custody.

The Crown Prosecution Service has its own guidelines for deciding whether it is in the public interest to proceed with a prosecution or whether diversion from the criminal justice system is appropriate. If the matter is dealt with at a Crown Court, it will be for a jury to decide whether the defendant is fit to plead, or whether they are too mentally disordered to stand trial. The judgement of fitness to plead includes consideration of whether the defendant understands the charge against them, whether they can meaningfully plead guilty or not guilty, and whether they have the capacity to instruct their legal representatives. In the past there has been concern that defendants who were unfit to plead and were then dealt with by compulsory admission to hospital, were implicitly being treated as if they were guilty. This situation has been progressively modified by the Criminal Procedure (Insanity) Act 1964, the Criminal Procedure (Insanity and Unfitness to Plead) Act 1991 and the Domestic Violence, Crime and Victims Act 2004. There now has to be a hearing of the facts of the case and the court then has three options: absolute discharge, a supervision order or a hospital order under the 1983 Mental Health Act.

Numerous disposals are available to the courts in criminal cases where it is found that a person was experiencing a mental disorder at the time they committed a crime. An order might be made under Section 37 of the 1983 Mental Health Act, which has the same effect as a Section 3 treatment order. This means that responsibility for the treatment and eventual discharge from section is under the jurisdiction of the responsible clinician. If the individual is deemed by the court to present a significant risk to the public, and usually where a serious offence against the person is involved, then a restriction order under Section 41 might also be made. This is usually made without restriction of time, and discharge from hospital can only be directed by the Home Secretary, or by a tribunal chaired by a member of the judiciary of at least equivalent standing to the judge who made the restriction order. As with tribunals in relation to civil sections of the 1983 Mental Health Act, there will be a requirement for a social circumstances report. A patient conditionally discharged under a restriction order is also likely to be liable to supervision in the community under a psychiatrist and 'social supervisor', a probation officer or social worker. This is a highly responsible area of practice, only undertaken by experienced workers, as the supervisor needs to be prepared to act promptly to affect a recall to hospital where circumstances are breaking down in the community and treatment in hospital is warranted.

Occasionally, prisoners are transferred to hospital under the 1983 Mental Health Act for treatment, and returned to prison to complete their sentence when they are considered to be sufficiently well. There are controversial cases where individuals are transferred to hospital towards the end of their sentence because they are deemed too dangerous and mentally disordered to return to the community – the 'One Flew Over The Cuckoo's Nest' scenario where the person then becomes detained beyond the end of their sentence. Individuals caught up in these circumstances are likely to feel that their continuing detention on an indefinite basis is contrary to natural justice. Mental health social workers who are involved in the preparation of such individuals for return to the community are likely to find them suspicious of authority because of their own perception that they have been dealt with unfairly.

Social work in secure mental health settings

Social workers who develop a specialty in working in forensic psychiatry may decide to move towards employment in secure mental health settings. Depending on their assessed level of dangerousness to others (and sometimes to themselves), patients may be placed in facilities which exist on a continuum of degree of security. At the highest level of security are the high security hospitals, Broadmoor, Rampton and Ashworth for England and Wales, and Carstairs for Scotland. To the visitor, these hospitals have the appearance of prisons with uniformed staff as warders. In fact the uniformed staff are all nurses, although membership of the Prison Officers' Association as their trade union has sometimes created ambiguity about their professional ethos. Despite the high level of perimeter security, the special hospitals have always sought to maintain a balance between containment and provision of a therapeutic regime. The popular perception is that people enter the special hospitals never to re-appear, but the average length of stay at Broadmoor is between six and seven years, although some individuals who continue to be considered dangerous accordingly can remain much longer (Sainsbury Centre for Mental Health 2006). Although the special hospitals are a national resource, there is some attempt to place patients in the hospital closest to their home to try to support relationships with families.

At medium levels of security are the regional secure units, smaller than the special hospitals, and with relatively lower levels of security, but still with perimeter fences, high staff to patient ratios, and locked wards. The patients placed in these units may be moving in one of two directions: for some it is a move from a special hospital towards further rehabilitation and subsequent discharge into the community, others may have been non-offenders whose behaviour was too challenging to be managed within low security settings, and who have been admitted for treatment until they are sufficiently stable to return to more open conditions. Finally, there are low secure units and Psychiatric Intensive Care Units (PICUs), some of which are located in local mental hospitals, and there is a growing level of private provision of such units. Department of Health policy implementation guidance defines these facilities:

> Psychiatric intensive care is for patients compulsorily detained usually in secure conditions, who are in an acutely disturbed phase of a serious mental disorder. There is an associated loss of

capacity for self control, with a corresponding increase in risk, which does not enable their safe, therapeutic management and treatment in a general open acute ward.

(Department of Health 2002: 3)

At all these levels of security, social workers are employed as members of the multidisciplinary team. Working in secure environments produces particular challenges, not least the need to resist incorporation into organisational cultures that can be inward looking and defensive (Rogers and Curran 2004). Policy-makers have made some efforts to address this tendency. For many years social workers employed in the special hospital were employed directly by the Department of Health (and its predecessor the Department of Health and Social Security). Latterly they have been employed by the social services authorities local to the special hospital to counter the isolation of these practitioners from mainstream professional cultures.

The role and contribution of social workers in secure settings is similar to those located in any multidisciplinary mental health team, though inevitably with an emphasis on maintaining a relationship between the service user and their family and other significant networks in the community. These connections become vulnerable during the patient's stay in secure conditions, but are critical if a successful move back into the community is to be effected. As the patient moves towards readiness for a move to the community or a facility with lower security, the social worker becomes a key broker with service providers and funders (patients who have been placed in a national or regional resource remain dependent on their local Trust or local authority for funding of placements). The value of social work to patient welfare in secure facilities is explicitly endorsed in the guidance for low secure units and PICUs:

> Social workers should be actively involved in the provision of social work assessments, CPA meetings and links with the MDT [multidisciplinary team] on the closed ward. Social workers also have a role in helping longer-term patients maintain social ties to the wider community by encouraging appropriate visits and activities.

(Department of Health 2002: 8)

Key points

- A key driver in relation to mental health policy is political and media perceptions of risk and dangerousness, fuelled by high profile tragedies which create distortion in the public perception of the level of dangerousness presented by individuals with mental health problems.

- People with a mental disorder are at far greater risk to themselves from self-harm and suicide than they are to the general population. Social workers who suspect that a service user is contemplating suicide should intervene sensitively but directly to avert this eventuality.

- Overall, people with mental health problems present no higher level of risk to others than the general population, but there are some factors that require careful assessment which may then need decisive intervention. These factors include: the disinhibiting effects of substance misuse in combination with a mental disorder; the potential influence of command hallucinations on an individual's behaviour; paranoid delusions; expressions of lack of empathy for the pain of others, and depression that gives rise to feelings of nihilism.

* Social workers play a key role in the implementation of statutory powers under the 1983 and 2007 Mental Health Acts, particularly in their capacity as Approved Mental Health Professionals to make applications for compulsory admission to hospital, or for a community treatment order.

* Social workers are regularly called on to provide the social circumstances report that is presented to Mental Health Review Tribunals. This is an opportunity to ensure that social perspectives are considered in decision-making about the liberty of detained patients.

* Social work can make an important contribution to multidisciplinary working in secure mental health settings, particularly in maintaining the relationship of the detained person to family and other significant community networks, and in arranging a return to non-secure provision or the community.

Key reading

Jones, R. (2008) *Mental Health Act Manual*, 11th edn, London: Sweet and Maxwell.

Prins, H. (1999) *Will They Do It Again? Risk Assessment and Management in Criminal Justice and Psychiatry*, London: Routledge.

Webb, D. and Harris R. (eds) (1999) *Mentally Disordered Offenders: managing people nobody owns*, London: Routledge.

9 The future of mental health social work

By the end of this chapter you should have an understanding of:

- Implications of the New Ways of Working programme for mental health social work

- The place of social work in functional mental health teams

- The content of 'The Ten Essential Shared Capabilities' and their implications for multidisciplinary practice

- The need for the development of leadership in relation to mental health social work

- The skills that are relevant to working across organisational boundaries

- The challenges to the role of social work presented by the personalisation agenda

- The challenges of developing research capacity and research-mindedness in relation to mental health social work

- Arguments for engagement by social workers in mental health policy development.

Planning the mental health workforce – 'new ways of working'

This chapter looks at current trends in the delivery of social work in mental health contexts – the workforce implications, new team structures, implications of joined-up services, the personalisation agenda, the need to develop and use the knowledge base for mental health social work – all of which seem to present social work with both threats and opportunities (Gould 2006a). On the negative side, many social work practitioners feel that their expertise will be marginalised by the dominance of clinical professions within integrated structures; this anxiety came to be symbolised by the replacement of the Approved Social Worker by the generic concept of the Approved Mental Health Professional in the 2007 Mental Health Act, as discussed in Chapter 8. Many of the transformations have been taking place under the umbrella of the post-1997 New Labour government's modernisation agenda, a policy direction that has had uncertain implications for social work. A trio of Department of Health papers in 1998 created a platform for this development: *Modernising Health and Social Services* (Department of Health 1998a) made the case for better coordination of services through formal partnerships, more consultation with service users, and a stronger evidence-based approach in health and social care; *Modernising Social Services* (Department of Health 1998b) set out a new institutional architecture for the governance of social care, proposed the creation of a General Social Care Council to regulate the workforce and was ultimately to lead to the setting up of the Social Care Institute for Excellence (SCIE) to develop the knowledge base; and, finally, *Modernising Mental Health Services* (Department of Health 1998c) reinforced these modernisation themes but with specific reference to 'joined up' mental health services, developed in partnership with service users and carers, and with a comprehensive approach to service development and access.

Chapter 8

Much of the change that has been implemented since the late 1990s has been led by the National Institute for Mental Health England (NIMHE), originally a unit within the Department of Health's Modernization Agency, but subsequently relocated within the Care Services Improvement Partnership and, from April 2009, redesignated the National Mental Health Development Unit. NIMHE has taken a lead responsibility for mapping the changing roles within the mental health workforce, particularly within the context of integrated services. This work has been taken forward by NIMHE's National Workforce Action Team, which has produced a number of reports around the theme of 'new ways of working'. Its report, *Mental Health: New Ways of Working for Everyone* (Department of Health 2007b), emphasises the need to find a balance between the contribution of individual professions and the holistic approach made by integrated teams:

> All workers have a unique contribution to make. However, it is by working as a team – by supporting one another to challenge existing practices that do not meet the needs of users and carers – that the mental health service can be most effective. By valuing the skills and insights of all those involved in care planning, ensuring that those workers with lived experience of mental distress play a significant role, every aspect of a person's life can be supported.
>
> (Department of Health 2007b: 6)

The New Ways of Working (NWW) programme has developed alongside the 'capable teams approach', a model for developing cohesive team practice based on 'a clear and simple five-step approach with a defined workforce focus, developed to support the integration of NWW and the new roles into the structures and practices of a multidisciplinary team, within existing resources' (Department of Health 2007b: 27). The five steps are: preparation and ownership; analysis of team function; identifying service user and carer needs; creating a needs-led workforce; and implementation and review. The approach was designed to be used in all areas of mental health, across health and social care, for all ages, in statutory, voluntary and private sectors, including all staff disciplines. The process helps a team reflect on their function, the needs of service users and carers, the current workforce structure and the current and required capabilities. The team's progress is recorded on a team profile and workforce plan, which feeds into the organisation's workforce planning process.

'New Ways of Working' emphasises the importance of the contribution of social work to the modernisation of mental health services, and in particular points to its progressive contribution to values-based practice:

> Social work makes an important contribution to mental health services and is a crucial component in their development. Social work values, skills and knowledge already encompass the approach set out in current government policy documents. These all emphasise the need for service users to participate actively in their care. Social workers have historically sought to work together with service users and their carers in partnership. More than any other profession, their value base is most closely aligned to this approach.
>
> (Department of Health 2007b: 117)

Social work and mental health teams

We have seen that social factors figure largely in the experience of mental distress and that the profession of social work has a significant role to play in the amelioration of that distress. Whether practitioners are located in specialist mental health agencies, or with other specialisms such as children's or adult services, mental health problems are presented by users of services across the life cycle. However, for social workers who work in adult mental health services times have been changing. The National Service Framework for Mental Health Services (Department of Health 1999) established a rationale for the reconfiguration of teams that was then given statutory force by the NHS Plan

(Department of Health 2000), giving guidance for the development and operation of community mental health teams, crisis resolution teams, assertive outreach teams and early intervention teams.

The core organisational unit of adult mental health services has for a number of years been the Community Mental Health Team (CMHT), comprising psychiatrists, psychologists, community psychiatric nurses, social workers and sometimes ancillary professions such as occupational health therapists. The National Service Framework diversified this provision with the creation of specialist, so-called 'functional' teams. The following descriptions of the role of functional teams are taken from the Department of Health's *Mental Health Policy Implementation Guide* (Department of Health 2001), a service development guideline that addresses implementation of the NHS National Plan.

Crisis resolution teams

Crisis resolution and home treatment teams are expected to:

- act as a 'gatekeeper' to mental health services, rapidly assessing individuals with acute mental health problems and referring them to the most appropriate service;

- provide immediate, multidisciplinary, community-based treatment twenty-four hours a day, seven days a week for individuals with severe, acute mental health problems for whom home treatment would be suitable;

- ensure that individuals experiencing severe, acute mental health difficulties are treated in the least restrictive environment as close to home as clinically possible;

- remain with the client until the crisis has resolved and the service user is linked with on-going care;

- if hospitalisation is necessary, be involved in discharge planning and provide intensive care at home to enable early discharge;

- reduce service users' vulnerability to crisis and maximise their vulnerability.

(Department of Health 2001: 11–12)

Assertive outreach teams

Assertive outreach teams are expected to carry relatively small caseloads and seek to engage individuals with severe and persistent mental disorders in accepting services. The teams are expected to:

- develop meaningful engagement with service users, provide evidence-based interventions and promote recovery;

- increase stability within the service users' lives, facilitate personal growth and provide opportunities for personal fulfilment;

- provide a service that is sensitive and responsive to service users' cultural, religious and gender needs;

- support the service user and his/her family/carers for sustained periods;

- promote effective interagency working;

- ensure effective risk assessment and management.

(Department of Health 2001: 26–27)

Early intervention teams

Early intervention teams are specifically intended to intervene with young people who appear to be developing the first episode of a psychosis, based on the evidence that this reduces the duration and severity of their disorder. Early intervention teams are expected to:

- reduce the stigma associated with psychosis and improve professional and lay awareness of the symptoms of psychosis and the need for early assessment;

- reduce the length of time young people remain undiagnosed and untreated;

- develop meaningful engagement, provide evidence-based interventions and promote recovery during the early phase of the illness;

- increase stability in the lives of service users, facilitate development and provide opportunities for personal fulfilment;

- provide a user-centred service, that is, a seamless service available for those from age 14 to 35 that effectively integrates child, adolescent and adult mental health services and works in partnership with primary care, education, social services, youth and other services;

- at the end of the treatment periods, ensure that the care is transferred thoughtfully and effectively.

(Department of Health 2001: 43–44)

The establishment of these functional teams has generally been viewed as a positive step in service development, and they have been seen as one of the markers of 'modernised' mental health services (Thornicroft and Tansella 2004), although the evidence for their effectiveness measured by outcomes for service users is contested. Burns and Lloyd (2004) reviewed the research in this area and concluded that the creation of functional teams was largely an act of faith based on little robust evidence that they improved outcomes for service users. They did report that one of the key factors in reducing admission to hospitals was the integration of social care into mental health services, although there was little evaluation of which models of integration were most likely to produce this outcome. Other psychiatrists have argued that the creation of functional multidisciplinary teams is part of an insidious erosion of the authority of the medical model in psychiatry (Craddock et al., 2008).

Social work and 'The Ten Essential Shared Capabilities'

One approach to identifying the roles of practitioners within multidisciplinary team settings is to map out the generic competencies or 'capabilities' that should be demonstrated by everyone. An influential approach to this in the British context has been 'The Ten Essential Shared Capabilities' (Hope 2004), an attempt to map out, or make explicit, that which should be embedded in the pre-qualifying training of all mental health professionals in order to deliver the objectives of the National Service framework for Mental Health and the NHS National Plan. The 'Capabilities' statement built on a report by The Sainsbury Centre for Mental Health (2001), and was then promoted by the Department of Health (see Box 9.1).

Box 9.1   The Ten Essential Shared Capabilities

- *Working in Partnership*. Developing and maintaining constructive working relationships with service users, carers, families, colleagues, lay people and wider community networks. Working positively with any tensions created by conflicts of interest or aspiration that may arise between the partners in care.

- *Respecting Diversity*. Working in partnership with service users, carers, families and colleagues to provide care and interventions that not only make a positive difference but also do so in ways that respect and value diversity including age, race, culture, disability, gender, spirituality and sexuality.

- *Practising Ethically*. Recognising the rights and aspirations of service users and their families, acknowledging power differentials and minimising them whenever possible. Providing treatment and care that is accountable to service users and carers within the boundaries prescribed by national (professional), legal and local codes of ethical practice.

- *Challenging Inequality*. Addressing the causes and consequences of stigma, discrimination, social inequality and exclusion on service users, carers and mental health services. Creating, developing or maintaining valued social roles for people in the communities they come from.

- *Promoting Recovery*. Working in partnership to provide care and treatment that enables service users and carers to tackle mental health problems with hope and optimism and to work towards a valued lifestyle within and beyond the limits of any mental health problem.

- *Identifying People's Needs and Strengths*. Working in partnership to gather information to agree health and social care needs in the context of the preferred lifestyle and aspirations of service users their families, carers and friends.

- *Providing Service User Centred Care.* Negotiating achievable and meaningful goals; primarily from the perspective of service users and their families. Influencing and seeking the means to achieve these goals and clarifying the responsibilities of the people who will provide any help that is needed, including systematically evaluating outcomes and achievements.

- *Making a Difference.* Facilitating access to and delivering the best quality, evidence-based, values-based health and social care interventions to meet the needs and aspirations of service users and their families and carers.

- *Promoting Safety and Positive Risk Taking.* Empowering the person to decide the level of risk they are prepared to take with their health and safety. This includes working with the tension between promoting safety and positive risk taking, including assessing and dealing with possible risks for service users, carers, family members and the wider public.

- *Personal Development and Learning.* Keeping up to date with changes in practice and participating in lifelong learning, personal and professional development for one's self and colleagues through supervision, appraisal and reflective practice.

From *The Ten Essential Shared Capabilities* (Hope 2004: 3)

For social workers these capabilities are fairly non-contentious, and reflect many of the values and principles of good practice. The overall approach of identifying generic core competencies as a basis for practice is not without critics: the assumption that all team members can all have the same transferable skills, and that professional background is relatively unimportant only seems to be promoted in the UK context. There is a lack of clarity about how these capabilities deliver better specified outcomes for service users or research to support this claim (Freeth et al., 2002; Zwarenstein et al., 2002). The converse view would be that the complexity of service user needs means that these cannot be met by a generic practitioner and will require collaborative teamwork delivered by practitioners with their own specialist knowledge and skills (Walsh et al., 2005).

Activity 9.1 Linking social work and the ten essential shared capabilities

Read Box 9.1 outlining The Ten Essential Shared Capabilities and consider how they relate to social work knowledge, values and skills.

- Which of the capabilities are social workers well prepared to demonstrate, and which would need to be augmented by additional learning?

- What kinds of outcomes for service users and carers might be improved by embedding The Ten Essential Shared Capabilities within team practice?

- Do social workers have additional capabilities that are not captured by The Ten Essential Shared Capabilities, and how do these contribute to the well-being of service users and carers?

Leadership

The anxiety for some social workers in integrated health and social care settings is the marginalisation of social work as a profession represented at managerial and supervisory levels. This may result in social workers being supervised by professionals from other backgrounds such as nursing, psychology or psychiatry and, at Trust level, executive managers who similarly are non-social work trained. Of course a competence-based approach such as 'The Ten Essential Shared Capabilities' would stress the generic commonalities of these occupations, but nevertheless there is anxiety that social work will lose ground, and have less capacity to influence services towards adopting social perspectives. These concerns underline the need for social work to build its capacity for leadership within mental health service structures as well as developing confidence in its professional authority. Indeed, research from the United States comparing the effectiveness of leadership of mental health teams found that social workers were particularly effective compared to other professions, not least because they had a democratic, facilitative leadership style that supported positive team functioning (Wells et al., 2006).

The development of leadership also involves the creation of a cadre of advanced practitioners. There is now a post-qualifying (PQ) framework, established by the General Social Care Council in England that establishes a pathway from qualifying to advanced practice in mental health (General Social Care Council 2007). The PQ framework is designed to be relevant to the education and training needs of all qualified social workers, including those in mental health and to complement and support regional and local workforce planning and development. The revised PQ Framework has a strong inter-professional orientation which potentially enables social workers and other professionals to study alongside one another. It will also ensure that all social workers have a strong grounding in inter-professional and inter-agency working while simultaneously developing their social work professionalism. Some NHS Trusts are already looking to develop multi-disciplinary training at a post-graduate diploma level.

Chapter 8

Although sections of the social work profession resisted the reform under the 2007 Mental Health Act of the Approved Social Worker role, to make it available to ancillary professionals under the title of Approved Mental Health Professionals (see Chapter 8), this legislation has also created opportunities for social work to assume lead clinical roles. Specifically, the newly created designation of Approved Clinician is available to social workers. The Approved Clinician acts as the responsible clinician for patients detained under the 1983 Mental Health Act, or subject to a guardianship order or community treatment order. This level of responsibility had previously been a monopoly held by psychiatrists (the Responsible Medical Officer under previous legislation) but the 2007 Act creates an opportunity for social workers and other professionals to assume this function. As Webber (2008) has commented, this may well be a developmental opportunity for practitioners who are operating at an advanced level, such as Consultant Social Workers, and potentially redresses some of the power of medical psychiatry.

There have also been a number of national and local initiatives designed to promote the awareness of leadership as an issue for the mental health social work workforce, and to stimulate capacity-building for leadership. This has included the joint creation of 'learning sets' by the National Institute for Mental Health England and Social Care Institute for England to support leadership development for the holders of key roles in social work and social care.

Working across boundaries

A recurring theme of this book has been the need for mental health social workers to adapt to working within integrated health and social care services. Depending on the degree of integration, and the rate at which services are moving along a continuum of integration, social workers may find that the service within which they are located is like a collectivity of smaller, partially integrated organisations. Sometimes an indicator of this state of partial integration is the existence of separate information technology systems, or distinct lines of accountability between health and social care personnel. Operating effectively in this environment requires well-honed skills of working across semi-permeable organisational boundaries, despite the outward public appearance of an integrated partnership Trust. At the same time the wider context of practice, incorporating the separation of commissioning and providing of services and the development of personalisation, where care may be purchased from a wide diversity of providers, also requires social workers to operate effectively in working between and across organisational boundaries (Bogg 2008). A key aspect of this shift from state monopoly to a mixed economy of care has been the transfer of much service provision to the voluntary and private sectors, requiring partnership working with these agencies to provide service users and carers with packages of care that meet their needs.

Chapter 1

One influential publication on the emergence of 'new' social models in mental health, discussed in Chapter 1, describes partnership as the 'lynchpin' of this development (Duggan et al., 2002). Duggan et al. identify the skills and knowledge-base of working within this networked mental health environment as:

- understanding of social structures, institutions and systems;
- awareness of the impact of multi-sectoral decisions on the lives of individuals and communities;
- commitment to strengthening the capacity of individuals, families, groups and communities;
- awareness of strategies for building community and individual capacity;

- willingness to challenge developments or practices that are not in the interests of individuals and communities or to empower and support individuals and communities to speak for themselves.

They comment that:

> These skills are the essence of the social approach and have particular relevance to mental health services. Moreover, as discussed here, it is clear that they are fundamental to the practice of all mental health professionals – not just those associated with social care.
>
> (Duggan et al., 2002: 7)

Despite the general consensus that partnership working is important in order to deliver joined-up, needs-led mental health services, there is still very little in the way of a rigorous evidence-base to sign-post which ways of working produce the best outcomes for service users and carers (Social Perspectives Network 2004; Brown and Cullis 2006). Nevertheless, there are some principles that can be iterated for effective working across boundaries and building partnerships (Buchanan and Carnwell 2005). These include the necessity to invest time and commitment to building inter-organisational relationships, including face-to-face contact, rather than assuming they can spontaneously emerge. The boundaries of partnership and joint working need to be made explicit both at strategic and operational levels, not least so that organisations feel confident that they can maintain their own sense of identity. Inter-organisational work operates within a context of inequalities of status and resources; small voluntary organisations and those led by service users and carers will be rightly concerned that cooperation will lead towards assimilation and control by budget-holding statutory agencies. Not least, there are critical issues in relation to information sharing, particularly in relation to data concerning individual service users. Different professions and sectors have their own cultures in relation to information-sharing, often supported by professional codes of practice and statutory requirements in relation to data protection, and ways of working need to evolve which respect these sensitivities.

Working with service users and carers – the challenge to professional identity

One key dimension to partnership working cited by Buchanan and Carnwell (2005) is the need to involve service users actively and to listen to their views (and carers should be added to this injunction). This is also underlined by the message from policy-makers that there is no rowing back from the personalisation agenda, that this will become 'mainstream' in professional practice and that prac-titioners will need to learn new skills (Carr 2008). Although, as was discussed earlier in this book, implementation of the constituent elements of the personalisation agenda – direct payments, indi-vidual budgets, personal budgets – has been more 'sticky' in mental health than in other areas of adult care (Carr 2008), the strong probabilities are that incrementally these reforms will also transform mental health care (notwithstanding the anxieties of critics who predict that those with the greatest impairments and highest levels of social inclusion will be further marginalised by this process).

In terms of skills for mental health social work this means building on core principles and values:

- a preventative approach

- the ability to work with complex situations and with different agencies and sectors

- the capacity to perform a wide range of tasks including brokerage and advocacy

- flexibility to step outside agency boundaries to serve people's best interests yet with the security of working in a regulated profession within a framework of law and regulation where people are accountable for their practice.

(Carr 2008)

And blending a range of roles and skills such as:

- advisers: helping clients to self-assess their needs and plan for their future care

- navigators: helping clients find their way to the service they want

- brokers: helping clients assemble the right ingredients for their care package from a variety of sources

- service providers: deploying therapeutic and counselling skills directly with clients risk assessors and auditors; especially in complex cases and with vulnerable people deemed to be a risk to themselves or other people

- designers of social care systems as a whole: to help draw together formal, informal, voluntary and private sector providers.

(Leadbeater et al., 2008)

As well as extending the traditional skills of mental health social workers, the personalisation agenda also reframes the conventional understandings of professional status, involving what one commentator has referred to as the 'death of deference' (Davis 2008). Sociologists of the professions used to characterise the professions as being defined by their legally protected title, university-based training, self-regulation, or by the processes by which they exert monopolistic control of specific functions. Increasingly, social work has been characterised as part of the 'new professionalism', where legitimacy derives not from the traditional sources of status – as in law and medicine – but from more democratic accountability to service users and carers and from values located in empowerment and participation (Hugman1991). It is not new for social work to engage with forms of practice that acknowledge that people are experts in their own problems – and this has echoes with early social work theories that advocated 'starting where the client is', but personalisation gives these perspectives statutory and formal authority. Mental health social workers will need to balance the tensions between these new forms of accountability which cede power to service users and carers, and forms of practice that prioritise risk management and control.

Building the knowledge base

We have already considered several of the challenges for social workers practising in a multidisciplinary environment. An additional aspect of this developing context of practice is the emphasis on 'evidence-based practice', first in medicine but now across many of the clinical professions. Here we usually are referring directly or indirectly to the approach developed by Sackett and others, claiming that evidence-based practice provides 'the conscientious, explicit and judicious use of the current best evidence in making decisions about the care of individual patients' (Sackett cited Tanenbaum 2003: 288). Social workers can feel marginalised by this trend because their profession has tended, in the words of Webber, to locate practice in, 'theoretical schema rather than empirical research' (Webber 2008: 1). Social work has also traditionally, particularly outside of the United States, been cautious about adopting approaches which privilege so-called positivism over the more inclusive approach to knowledge which accepts as legitimate those forms of evidence which are located in practice and subjective experience. One consequence of this has been the preference of broader terms such as knowledge-based or knowledge-informed practice rather than 'evidence-based'.

Some of this controversy has centred around the adherence of evidence-based medicine to a hierarchical view of what constitutes the best evidence to guide practice, ordered in a hierarchy which places at its apex the systematic reviews of randomised controlled trials (RCTs), descending through single RCTs, quasi-experimental studies, qualitative research and, finally, clinical expertise. This approach, which takes the RCT to be the gold standard for evidence, and downgrades practitioner knowledge and virtually excludes the voice of service users and carers, has been particularly controversial for social work, and has led to various efforts to propose more pluralistic, non-hierarchical approaches to identifying knowledge to guide practice (Pawson et al., 2003; Gould 2006b). It has also provoked academics, practitioners and service user researchers to attempt to articulate approaches to doing and using research in mental health that are values-based rather than driven solely by methodological priorities (Tew et al., 2006).

Some of this discourse around social work knowledge and evidence-based practice tends to be defensive, as well as overlooking the debates within evidence-based psychiatry itself, which show that there is an awareness of the potential narrowness of orthodox evidence-based medicine (e.g., Burns and Catty 2002; Marshall 2002; Cooper 2003). Social work, including mental health social work, has a more extensive and significant body of research evidence available to it than is often acknowledged, even from within the profession. If we start from the position that the form of evidence that is relevant for practitioners starts from the question that is being asked (e.g., 'How does it feel to have this experience?', 'What kind of intervention is most helpful for this group of service users?', 'How should we organise services to make this kind of support accessible?'), then social work has an extensive knowledge-base from which to draw (Gould 2006b; Gould 2008). Some of this evidence-base is woven throughout the content of this book.

This is not to be complacent. Research in mental health has tended to focus on answering questions that are amenable to answering categorically through experimental research designs such as randomised controlled trials, not least because these are most relevant to questions about drug effectiveness and to attract funding from pharmacological companies and other powerful interest groups (Rose 2007). A survey conducted by the author and colleagues of mental health practitioners, researchers, service users and carers identified areas where there is need for further research in order to guide practice (Gould et al., 2007). Overall, the survey demonstrated a significant level of interest in social research in mental health across a range of constituencies including professionals in both social care and health sectors, and among service users. This is encouraging, given the relatively low priority that has been given to social research in recent years within mental health research activity as a whole, or within social work as a disciplinary area (Huxley 2001; Huxley 2002). The clearest indication from the survey was the emergent consensus across a wide cross-section of interests, that *social inclusion/ social capital/social networks* and *social factors that enable resilience and recovery* were the highest priority topics for research. This resonates with the themes of this book that mental health social work needs to engage with and draw from research on the social context of practice.

The other side of the equation of evidence-based mental health social work – the production of relevant knowledge – is the need to develop the overall research capacity of the mental health social work workforce. This involves developmental activity on a number of fronts in order to enhance social work research capacity in mental health and, in turn, contribute to practitioner confidence and role clarity in integrated services. This includes building on the existing achievements of service user researchers in initiating and leading research collaborations, focusing efforts to build research minded-ness among social work and social care practitioners through qualifying and post-qualifying education, mentoring practitioner researchers, creating senior social research positions in service organisations, building partnerships between universities and providers, and creating fellowships to foster the recruitment and training of career researchers (Gould et al., 2007).

Promoting social perspectives and policy

An underpinning argument of this book has been that mental health social workers need to be able to locate their practice within a wider social and political context (and that – reciprocally – their practice will be influenced by those contextual understandings). As Bracken and Thomas have argued, 'it is important to recognise the negative effect that noxious social environments have on mental health' (2005: 266). This leads to their view that there is an overlap between mental health practice, 'and community action aimed at increasing social cohesion, building on social capital, and struggling against social inequality and oppression'. This perspective is fundamental to defining social work's role and purpose, as enshrined in the definition held jointly by the International Federation of Social Workers and International Association of Schools of Social Work, cited in the British Association of Social Workers' code of ethics:

> The social work profession promotes social change, problem solving in human relationships and the empowerment and liberation of people to enhance well-being. Utilising theories of human

behaviour and social systems, social work intervenes at the points where people interact with their environments. Principles of human rights and social justice are fundamental to social work.

(British Association of Social Workers, *Code of Ethics:*
http://www.basw.co.uk/Portals/0/CODE%20OF%20ETHICS.pdf)

The British Association of Social Workers' code of ethics upholds as a duty of social workers the use of professional knowledge and experience to contribute to the development of social policy. Social workers have been prominent in the campaigns to influence mental health legislation and the new social models in mental health reinforce the importance of the profession's engagement in 'not only civil and political but also economic, social and cultural rights' (BASW Code of Ethics). Although mental health social workers can feel overwhelmed by workloads and expectations placed upon them, seeking wherever it is possible to influence the mental health policy environment towards social perspectives should not be overlooked.

Conclusion

Social work brings skills, knowledge and values to the delivery of services to people who are in mental distress. Alone within the multidisciplinary environment of modern mental health services social workers have a professional education that is grounded in social sciences, the law in relation to vulnerable adults and children, knowledge of social care services for people across the life-cycle, and a value base that emphasises anti-discrimination and anti-oppression. Mental health social work faces many challenges that include recruitment and retention of newly qualified practitioners to its ranks, and the building of confidence and expertise to sustain its distinct voice within medically dominated multidisciplinary contexts. To repeat – but complete – the quotation with which this book opened:

Social work and social workers are important. Social work makes an important contribution to mental health services and is a crucial component in their development. . . . However, like any other profession, social workers cannot afford to rest on their laurels and stand still. If they do, they will get left behind. In an increasingly rapidly changing world of new demands and pressures, where there is a need for a more flexible and well-trained workforce, it is vital that social workers fully embrace this culture shift and seize fresh opportunities, including New Ways of Working. This does not mean they should abandon their highly prized and well-recognised value base – far from it. They should continue to champion both their approach and their cause, but should do so in a positive and outward-looking way.

(Department of Health, 2007b: 117)

Key points

- The development of integrated mental health services places demands on all professions, including social workers, to develop new ways of working that are effective.

- A key aspect of the implementation of the New Service Framework for Mental Health Services is the creation of specialist 'functional' teams such as crisis resolution teams, early intervention teams and assertive outreach teams.

- One approach to supporting the integration of multidisciplinary mental health teams is through identification of generic competencies, notably 'The Ten Essential Shared Capabilities', although it is contested whether these lead to measurable improvement in service user outcomes.

- The identity of social work within integrated mental health services will depend upon the development of sufficient leadership capacity within the profession, and the creation of a cadre of advanced practitioners.

- The promotion of social perspectives within a mixed economy of mental health care also requires that social workers have the skills to work between and across organisational boundaries.

- The personalisation agenda challenges traditional conceptions of the professional as expert, and mental health social workers will have to adopt approaches that are sensitive to new forms of accountability to service users and carers.

- The effectiveness of mental health social work depends on the continuing development of research capacity, and the readiness of practitioners to engage in developing knowledge- or evidence-based practice.

- An important element of established definitions of social work, reinforced by professional codes of practice, is the willingness to engage in activities directed at influencing policy, including mental health policy.

Key reading

Department of Health (2007b) *Mental Health: New Ways of Working for Everyone*, London: Department of Health. Available as download from http://www.dh.gov.uk/en/Publicationsandstatistics/Publications/PublicationsPolicy AndGuidance/DH_079102

Onyett, S. (2003) *Teamworking in Mental Health*, Basingstoke: Palgrave Macmillan.

Webber, M. (2008) *Evidence-based Policy and Practice in Mental Health Social Work*, Exeter: Learning Matters.

Bibliography

Abramowitz, J.S. (2004) 'Treatment of obsessive-compulsive disorder in patients who have comorbid major depression', *Journal of Clinical Psychology*, 60: 1133–1141.

Adamson, J. (2001) 'Awareness and understanding of dementia in African/Caribbean and South Asian families', *Health and Social Care in the Community*, 9: 391–396.

Age Concern (2007) *Older People in the United Kingdom: key facts and statistics 2007*, London: Age Concern.

Aldridge, J. and Becker, S. (2003) *Children Caring for Parents with Mental Illness: perspectives of young carers, parents and professionals*, Bristol: Policy Press.

Allebeck, P. (1989) 'Schizophrenia: a life-shortening disease', *Psychiatric Bulletin*, 15: 81–89.

Allmark, P. (2002) 'Can there be an ethics of care?', in K. Fulford, D. Dickenson and T. Murray (eds) *Healthcare Ethics and Human Values*, Oxford: Blackwell.

Allott, P. and Loganathan, L. (2002) 'Discovering hope for recovery from a British perspective: a review of literature', Birmingham: Centre for Community Mental Health, University of Central England.

Alzheimer's Society (2007) *Dementia UK: The Full Report*, London: The Alzheimer's Society.

American Academy of Child and Adolescent Psychiatry (1997) 'Practice parameters for the assessment and treatment of children and adolescents with conduct disorder', *Journal of the American Academy of Child and Adolescent Psychiatry*, 36, Supplement 10: 122S–139.

American Diabetes Association, American Psychiatric Association, American Association of Clinical Endocrinologists, North American Association for the Study of Obesity (2004) 'Consensus development conference on antipsychotic drugs and obesity and diabetes', *Journal of Clinical Psychiatry*, 65: 267–272.

American Psychiatric Association (1994) *Diagnostic and Statistical Manual of Mental Disorder*, 4th edn, Washington: American Psychiatric Association.

Angold, A. and Costello, E. (2001) 'The epidemiology of depression in children and adolescents', in I. Goodyer (ed.) *The Depressed Child and Adolescent*, 2nd edn, Cambridge: Cambridge University Press.

Appleby, L., Shaw, J., Amos, T., McDonnell, R., Harris, C., McCann, K., Davies, C., Buckley, H. and Parsons, R. (1999) '"Suicide with 12 months off" contact with mental health services: national clinical survey', *British Medical Journal*, 318: 1235–1239.

Aston, J., Atkinson, J., Evans, C., Davis, S. and O'Regan, S. (2003) *Employers and the NDDP: Qualitative research first wave*, Sheffield: Institute for Employment Studies.

Atkinson, D. (1999) *Advocacy: a review*, York: Joseph Rowntree Foundation.

Audit Commission (1986) *Making A Reality of Community Care*, London: Audit Commission.

Baldwin, C. and Capstick, A. (eds) (2007) *Tom Kitwood on Dementia: a reader and critical commentary*, Maidenhead: Open University Press.

Baldwin, M. (2000) *Care Management and Community Care: social work discretion and the construction of policy*, Aldershot: Ashgate.

Barnes, C., Oliver, M. and Barton, L. (eds) (2002) *Disability Studies Today*, Cambridge: Polity.

Barnes, M. and Bowl, R. (2001) *Taking Over The Asylum: Empowerment and Mental Health*, Basingstoke: Palgrave.

Baron-Cohen, S. (2009) 'Media distortion damages both science and journalism', *New Scientist*, 2701: 26–27.

Baruch, G. and Treacher, A. (1978) *Psychiatry Observed*, London: Routledge.

Bateman, N. (1995) *Advocacy Skills*, Aldershot: Arena.

Beck, A. (1983) 'Cognitive theory of depression: new perspectives', in P. Clayton and J. Barret (eds) *Treatment of Depression: old controversies and new approaches*, New York: Raven Press.

Beck, A. (1996) *Beck Depression Inventory*, San Antonio: The Psychological Corporation.

Beck, A., Rush, A., Shaw, B. and Emery, G. (1979) *Cognitive Therapy for Depression*, New York: Guilford Press.

Beck, U. (1992) *Risk Society: Towards a New Modernity*, London: Sage Publications.

Beddington, J., Cooper, C., Field, J., Goswami, U., Hupert, F., Jenkins, J., Kirkwood, T., Sahakian, B. and Thomas, S. (2008) 'The mental wealth of nations', *Nature*, 455: 1057–1060.

Beresford, P. (2002) 'Thinking about "mental health": towards a social model', *Journal of Mental Health*, 11: 581–584.

Bentall, R. (2003) *Madness Explained: Psychosis and Human Nature*, London: Allen Lane.

Bhugra, D. and Bhui, K. (2001) 'African-Caribbeans and schizophrenia: contributing factors', *Advanced Psychiatric Treatment*, 7: 283–291.

Bianchetti, A., Scuratti, A., Zanetti, O., Binetti, G., Frisoni, G., Magni, E. and Trabucci, M. (1995) 'Predictors of mortality and institutionalization in Alzheimer disease patients 1 year after discharge from an Alzheimer dementia unit', *Dementia*, 6: 108–112.

Biestek, F. (1961) *The Casework Relationship*, London: Allen and Unwin.

Black, D., Baumgard, C., Bell, S. and Kao, C. (1996) 'Death rates in 71 men with antisocial personality disorder: a comparison with general population mortality', *Psychosomatics*, 37: 131–136.

Blanchard, E. and Hickling, E. (2004) *After the Crash. Psychological Assessment and Treatment of Survivors of Motor Vehicle Accidents*, 2nd edn, Washington, DC: APA.

Bogg, D. (2008) *The Integration of Mental Health Social Work and the NHS*, Exeter: Learning Matters.

Bourdieu, P. (1986) 'The forms of capital', in J. Richardson (ed.) *A Handbook of Theory and Research for the Sociology of Education*, New York: Greenwood.

Bracken, P. and Thomas, P. (2005) *Postpsychiatry: mental health in a postmodern world*, Oxford: Oxford University Press.

Breaky, W. (1996) 'Clinical work with homeless people in the USA', in D. Bhugra (ed.) *Homelessness and Mental Health: studies in social and community psychiatry*, Cambridge: Cambridge University Press.

British Association of Social Workers (2006) 'Briefing paper on the Mental Health Bill 2006'. Online: http://www.spn.org.uk/fileadmin/SPN_uploads/Documents/BASW_Parliamentary_briefing.rtf (accessed 10 May 2009).

Brodaty, H., Green, A. and Koschera, A. (2003) 'Meta-analysis of psychosocial interventions for caregivers of people with dementia', *Journal of the American Geriatrics Society*, 14: 936–940.

Brooker, D. (2001) 'Therapeutic Activity', in C. Cantley (ed.) *A Handbook of Dementia Care*, Buckingham: Open University Press.

Broverman, I., Broverman, D., Clarkson, F., Rosencrantz, P. and Vogel, S. (1970) 'Sex role stereotypes and clinical judgements of mental health', *Journal of Consulting and Clinical Psychology*, 34: 1–7.

Brown, G. and Harris, T. (1978) *The Social Origins of Depression*, London: Tavistock.

Brown, G. and Rutter, M. (1966) 'The measurement of family activities and relationships: a methodological study', *Human Relations*, 19: 241–263.

Brown, G., Monck, E., Carstairs, G. and Wing, J. (1962) 'Influence of family life on the course of schizophrenic illness', *British Journal of Preventive and Social Medicine*, 16: 55–68.

Brown, G., Andrews, B., Harris, T., Adler, Z. and Bridge, L. (1986) 'Social support, self-esteem and depression', *Psychological Medicine*, 19: 813–831.

Brown, L. and Cullis, J. (2006) 'Team production and policy for the care of older people: problems with theory and evidence', *Policy Studies*, 27: 55–69.

Brown, S. (1997) 'Excess mortality of schizophrenia. A meta-analysis', *British Journal of Psychiatry*, 171: 502–508.

Buchanan, J. and Carnwell, R. (2005) 'Developing best practice in partnership', in R. Carnwell and J. Buchanan (eds) *Effective Practice in Health and Social Care: A Partnership Approach*, Maidenhead: Open University Press.

Burchardt, T. (2000) 'Social exclusion' in M. Davies (ed.) *The Blackwell Encyclopaedia of Social Work*, Oxford: Blackwell.

Burchardt, T. (2003) *Employment Retention and the Onset of Sickness or Disability: evidence from Labour Force Survey longitudinal datsets. DWP In-house report 109*, London: HMSO.

Burchardt, T., LeGrand, J. and Piachaud, D. (2002) 'Degrees of exclusion: developing a dynamic, multidimensional measure', in J. Hills, J. LeGrand and D. Piachaud (eds) *Understanding Social Exclusion*, Oxford: Oxford University Press.

Burns, T. and Catty, J. (2002) 'Mental health policy and evidence', *Psychiatric Bulletin*, 26: 324–327.

Burns, T. and Lloyd, H. (2004) 'Is a team approach based on staff meetings cost-effective in the delivery of mental health care?', *Current Opinion in Psychiatry*, 17: 311–314.

Burr, V. (1995) *Social Constructivism*, London: Routledge.

Burton, N. (2006) *Psychiatry*, Oxford: Blackwell.

Butler, I. and Drakeford, M. (2005) *Scandal, Social Policy and Welfare*, 2nd edn, Bristol: Policy Press.

Cameron, M., Edmans, T., Greatley, A. and Morris, D. (2003) *Community Renewal and Mental Health*, London: King's Fund.

CAMHS Review (2008) *Improving the Mental Health and Psychological Well-being of Children and Young People: National CAMHS Review interim report*, London: Children and Mental Health Services Review.

Campbell, T. and Heginbotham, C. (1991) *Mental Illness, Prejudice and the Law*, Aldershot: Dartmouth.

Cantley, C. (ed.) (2001) *A Handbook of Dementia Care*, Buckingham: Open University Press.

Cantor-Graae, E. and Selten, J. (2005) 'Schizophrenia and migration: a meta-analysis and review', *American Journal of Psychiatry*, 162: 12–24.

Care Services Improvement Partnership, Royal College of Psychiatrists and Social Care Institute for Excellence (2007) *A Common Purpose: recovery in future mental health services, Joint position paper 08*, London: Social Care Institute for Excellence.

Carnwell, R. and Buchanan, J. (eds) (2005) *Effective Practice in Health and Social Care: a partnership approach*, Maidenhead: Open University Press.

Carr, A. (1999) *The Hand Report of Child and Adolescent Clinical Psychology: a contextual approach*, London: Routledge.

Carr, S. (2008) *SCIE Report 20: Personalisation: A Rough Guide*, London: Social Care Institute for Excellence.

Carr, S. and Robbins, D. (2009) *Research Briefing 20: The implementation of individual budget schemes in adult social care*, London: Social Care Institute for Excellence.

Cassano, P. and Fava, M. (2002) 'Depression and public health: An overview', *Journal of Psychosomatic Research*, 53: 849–857.

Challis, D., Chessum, R., Chesterman, J., Luckett, R. and Traske, K. (1990) *Case Management in Social and Health Care: the Gateshead Community Care Scheme*, Canterbury: Personal Social Services Research Unit.

Chen, E., Harrison, G. and Standen, P. (1991) 'Management of first episode psychotic illness in Afro-Caribbean patients', *British Journal of Psychiatry*, 158: 517–522.

Cheston, R. and Bender, M. (1999) *Understanding Dementia: the man with the worried eyes*, London: Jessica Kingsley.

Chilvers, R., Macdonald, G. and Hayes, A. (2006) 'Supported housing for people with severe mental disorders', *Cochrane Database of Systematic Reviews, 2006*, Issue 4: Art. No.: CD000453. DOI:10.1002/14651858. CD000453.pub2.

Churchill, R. (2007) *International Experiences of Using Community Treatment Orders*, Institute of Psychiatry, Kings College London. Online: http://www.iop.kcl.ac.uk/news/downloads/final2ctoreport8march07.pdf (accessed 10 June 2009).

Citizens Advice Bureau (2004) *Out of the Picture: CAB evidence on mental health and social exclusion*, London: CAB.

Clare, A. (1977) *Psychiatry in Dissent: controversial issues in thought and practice*, 2nd edn, London: Tavistock Publications.

Cohen, S. (1987) *Folk Devils and Moral Panics: the creation of the mods and rockers*, 2nd edn, Oxford: Blackwell.

Coid, J., Min Yang, M., Roberts, A. and Ullrich, S. (2006) 'Prevalence and Correlates of Personality Disorder in Great Britain', *British Journal of Psychiatry*, 188: 423–431.

Cole, M.G., Bellavance, F. and Mansour, A. (1999) 'Prognosis of depression in elderly community and primary care populations: a systematic review and meta-analysis', *American Journal of Psychiatry*, 156: 1182–1189.

Coleman, J. (1988) 'Social capital in the creation of human capital', *American Journal of Sociology*, 94 (supplement): S95–S120.

Commission for Healthcare Audit and Inspection (2007) *Count Me In 2007: results of the 2007 national census of inpatients in mental health and learning disability services in England and Wales*, London: Commission for Healthcare Audit and Inspection.

Cooper, B. (2003) 'Evidence-based mental health policy: a critical appraisal', *British Journal of Psychiatry*, 183: 105–112.

Corden, A. and Sainsbury, R. (2003) *Evaluation of the Disabled Person's Tax Credit: views and experiences of recipients. Social Policy Research Unit, Inland Revenue Research Report 5*. Online: http://www.inlandrevenue. gov.uk/research/report5-dptcqualitative.pdf (accessed 10 May 2009).

Corden, A., Nice, K. and Sainsbury, R. (2005) *Incapacity Benefit Reforms Pilot: findings from a longitudinal panel of clients, Department of Work and Pensions, Research Report No 259*, London: Department of Work and Pensions.

Costello, J., Compton, S., Keeler, G. and Angold, A. (2003) 'Relationships between poverty and psychopathology: a natural experiment', *JAMA*, 290: 2023–2029.

Coultard, M., Farrell, M., Singleton, N. and Meltzer, H. (2000) *Tobacco, Alcohol and Drug Use and Mental Health*, London: The Stationery Office.

Craddock, N. and Jones, I. (1999) 'Genetics of bipolar disorder', *Journal of Medical Genetics*, 36: 585–594.

Craddock, N., Antebi, D., Attenburrow, M.-J., Bailey, A., Carson. A., Cowen. P. et al. (2008) 'Wake-up call for British psychiatry', *British Journal of Psychiatry*, 193: 6–9.

Crane, M. (1999) *Understanding Older Homeless People*, Buckingham: Open University Press.

Crook, F. (2007) 'Second thoughts: prisons are losing the mental illness battle', *The Guardian*, Wednesday 31 October 2007. Online: http://www.guardian.co.uk/society/2007/oct/31/guardiansocietysupplement.comment1 (accessed 8 May 2009).

Crowther, R., Marshal, M., Bond, G. and Huxley, P. (2004) 'Vocational rehabilitation for people with severe mental illness (Cochrane Review)', The Cochrane Library, Issue 3, 2006 (Reprint).

CSIP/NIMHE (undated) *Mental Health First Aid*, York: Care Services Improvement Partnership/National Institute for Mental Health in England.

CSIP/NIMHE (2007) *Mental Health: New Ways of Working for Everyone*, York: Care Services Improvement Partnership/National Institute for Mental Health England.

Cumming, E. and Henry, W. (1961) *Growing Old: the process of disengagement*, New York: Basic Books.

Cutler, T., Wain, B. and Behoney, K. (2007) 'A new epoch of individualization? Problems with the "personalization" of public sector services', *Public Administration*, 85: 847–855.

Davis, A. (2003) 'Mental health and personal finances – a literature review'. Unpublished paper for the Office of the Deputy Prime Minister Social Exclusion Unit.

Davis, R. (2008) 'Death of deference and its impact on social care', *Community Care*, 29 October 2008.

Dearden, C. and Becker, S. (1995) *Young Carers: the facts*, Loughborough: Young Carers Research Group.

Demott, K., Bick, D., Norman, R., Ritchie, G., Turnbull, N., Adams, C. et al. (2006) *Clinical Guidelines and Evidence Review for Post Natal Care: routine post natal care of recently delivered women and their babies*, London: National Collaborating Centre for Primary Care and Royal College Of General Practitioners.

Department for Children, Schools and Families (2004) *Every Child Matters*, London: Department for Children, Schools and Families.

Department of Health (1989) *Caring for People: community care in the next decade and beyond*, London: Department of Health.

Department of Health (1991) *The Care Programme Approach*, London: Department of Health.

Department of Health (1998a) *Modernising Health and Social Services*, London, Department of Health.

Department of Health (1998b) *Modernising Social Services*, London, Department of Health.

Department of Health (1998c) *Modernising Mental Health Services*, London, Department of Health.

Department of Health (1999) *Modern Standards and Service Models: national service framework for mental health*, London: The Stationery Office.

Department of Health (2000) *The NHS Plan. A plan for investment. A plan for reform*, London: Department of Health.

Department of Health (2001) *The Mental Health Policy Implementation Guide*, London: Department of Health.

Department of Health (2002) *National Minimum Standards for General Adult Services in Psychiatric Intensive Care Units (PICU) and Low Secure Environments*, London: Department of Health.

Department of Health (2004a) *Choosing Health: making healthy choices easier*, London: Department of Health.

Department of Health (2004b) *CAMHS Standard, National Service Framework for Children, Young People and Maternity Services*, London: Department of Health.

Department of Health (2005) *Independence, Well-being and Choice: our vision for the future of social care for adults in England, CM6499*, London: Department of Health.

Department of Health (2006a) *Our Health, Our Care, Our Say: a new direction for community services*, London: Department of Health.

Department of Health (2006b) *Transitions: getting it right for young people*, London: Department of Health.

Department of Health (2007a) *Capabilities for Inclusive Practice*, London: National Social Inclusion Programme.

Department of Health (2007b) *Mental Health: new ways of working for everyone*, London: Department of Health.

Department of Health (2007c) *Making the CPA Work for You*, London: Department of Health.

Department of Health (2007d) *Best Practice in Managing Risk: principles and guidance for best practice in the assessment and management of risk to self and others in mental health services*, London: Department of Health.

Department of Health (2008a) *Refocusing the Care Programme Approach: best practice guidance*, London: Department of Health.

Department of Health (2008b) *Improving Access to Psychological Therapies Implementation Plan: national guidelines for regional delivery*, London: Department of Health.

Department of Health and Social Security (1975) *Better Services for the Mentally Ill*, London: HMSO.

Desjarlais, R., Eisenberg, I., Good, B. and Kleinman, A. (1996) *World Mental Health: Problems and Priorities in Low Income Countries*, Oxford: Oxford University Press.

Dohrenwend, B. and Dohrenwend, B. (1977) 'Sex differences in mental illness: a reply to Gove and Tudor', *American Journal of Sociology*, 82: 1336–1341.

Donnelly, M. (1992) *The Politics of Mental Health in Italy*, London: Routledge.

Doyal, L. and Gough, I. (1991) *A Theory of Human Need*, Basingstoke: Macmillan.

Drake, R., Hugo, G., Bebort, R., Becker, D., Harris, M., Bond, G. and Quimby, E. (1999) 'A randomized clinical trial of supported employment for inner-city patients with severe mental disorders', *Archives of General Psychiatry*, 56: 627–633.

Duggan, C., Huband, N., Smailagic, N., Ferriter, M. and Adams, C. (2007) 'The use of psychological treatments for people with personality disorder: a systematic review of randomized controlled trials', *Personality and Mental Health*, 1: 95–125.

Duggan, M. with Cooper, A. and Foster, J. (2002) *Modernising the Social Model in Mental Health: a discussion paper*, London: Social Perspectives Network.

Dunn, S. (1999) *Creating Accepting Communities*, London: MIND.

Engel, G. (1980) 'The clinical application of the biopsychosocial model', *American Journal of Psychiatry*, 137: 535–544.

Erikson, E. (1977) *Childhood and Society*, London: Paladin.

Ethier, L.S., Lacharite, C. and Couture, G. (1995) 'Childhood adversity, parental stress and depression of negligent mothers', *Child Abuse and Neglect*, 19: 619–632.

Evans, O., Singleton, N., Meltzer, H., Stewart, R. and Prince, M. (2003) *The Mental Health of Older People*, London: Office for National Statistics.

Falkov, A. (1995) *Study of Working Together 'Part 8' Reports*, London: Department of Health.

Fawcett, B. and Karban, K. (2005) *Contemporary Mental Health: theory, policy and practice*, Oxon: Routledge.

Ferguson, I. (2007) 'Increasing user choice or privatizing risk? The antinomies of personalization', *British Journal of Social Work*, 37: 387–403.

Fernando, S. (1991) *Mental Health, Race and Culture*, London: Macmillan.

Ford, T., Goodman, R. and Meltzer, H. (2003) 'The British Child and Adolescent Mental Health Survey 1999: the prevalence of *DSM-IV* disorders', *Journal of the American Academy of Child and Adolescent Psychiatry*, 42: 1203–1211.

Foucault, M. (1961) *Madness and Civilization: a history of insanity in the age of reason*, London: Routledge.

Foulkes, S. (1983). *Introduction to Group-Analytic Psychotherapy: studies in the social integration of individuals and groups*, London: Maresfield Reprints.

Freeth, D., Hammick, M., Koppel, I., Reeves, S. and Barr, H. (2002) *A Critical Review of Evaluations for Interprofessional Education*, London: LTSN – Centre for Health Sciences and Practice.

Frick, P., Kamphaus, R., Lahey, B. Loeber, R., Christ, M., Hart, E. and Tannenbaum, L. (1991) 'Academic under-achievement and the disruptive behaviour disorders', *Journal of Consulting and Clinical Psychology*, 59: 289–294.

Fryers, T., Melzer, D. and Jenkins, R. (2003) 'Social inequalities and the common mental disorders: a systematic review of the evidence', *Social Psychiatry and Psychiatric Epidemiology*, 38: 229–237.

Gelder, M., Gath, D. and Mayou, R. (1983) *Oxford Textbook of Psychiatry*, Oxford: Oxford University Press.

General Social Care Council (2007) *Specialist Standards and Requirements for Post-qualifying Social Work Education and Training. Social work in mental health services*, London: General Social Care Council.

Giddens, A. (1991) *Modernity and Self Identity: self and society in the late modern age*, Stanford, CA: Stanford University Press.

Gigerenzer, G. (2002) *Reckoning With Risk: Learning To Live With Uncertainty*, London: Penguin.

Gilbert, P. (2003) *The Value of Everything: social work and its importance in the field of mental health*, Lyme Regis; Russell House.

Giles, D., Jarrett, R., Biggs, M., Guzick, D. and Rush, A. (1989) 'Clinical predictors of recurrence in depression', *American Journal of Psychiatry*, 146: 764–767.

Gilligan, C. (1982) *In a Different Voice: psychological theory and women's development*, Cambridge: Cambridge University Press.

Glasby, J. and Dickinson, H. (2008) *Partnership Working in Health and Social Care*, Bristol: Policy Press.

Glasby, J. and Peck, E. (2003) *Care Trusts: partnership working in action*, Abingdon: Radcliffe.

Godfrey, M., Townsend, J., Surr, C., Boyle, G. and Brooker, D. (2005) 'Prevention and Service Provision: mental health problems in later life – summary report to the Inquiry Board, the UK inquiry into mental health and well-being in later life'. Online: http://www.mhilli.org/documents/SummaryReporttotheEnquiryBoard.pdf (accessed 7 May 2009).

Goldberg, D. and Huxley, P. (1980) *Mental Illness in the Community: pathways to psychiatric care*, London: Tavistock.

Goldberg, D. and Huxley, P. (1992) *Common Mental Disorders: a bio-social model*, London: Tavistock/Routledge.

Goldberg, E. (1985) *Problems, Tasks and Outcomes: an evaluation of task centered casework in three settings*, London: Allen and Unwin.

Goodyer, I., Herbert, J., Tamplin, A. and Altham, P. (2000) 'First-episode major depression in adolescents. Affective, cognitive and endocrine characteristics of risk status and predictors of onset', *British Journal of Psychiatry*, 176: 142–149.

Gould, N. (2001) 'Familicide', in G. Howarth and O. Leaman (eds) *Encyclopaedia of Death and Dying*, London: Routledge.

Gould, N. (2005) 'International trends in mental health policy', in S. Quin and B. Redmond (eds) *Mental Health and Social Policy in Ireland*, Dublin: University College Dublin Press.

Gould, N. (2006a) 'Social inclusion as an agenda for mental health social work: getting a whole life?', *Journal of Policy Practice*, 5: 77–90.

Gould, N. (2006b) 'An inclusive approach to knowledge for mental health social work practice and policy', *British Journal of Social Work*, 36: 109–125.

Gould, N. (2006c) *Mental Health and Child Poverty*, York: Joseph Rowntree Foundation.

Gould, N. (2008) 'Research' in M. Davies (ed.) *The Blackwell Companion To Social Work*, Oxford: Blackwell.

Gould, N. and Kendall, T. (2007) 'Developing the NICE/SCIE guidelines for dementia care: the challenges of enhancing the evidence base for social and health care', *British Journal of Social Work*, 37: 475–490.

Gould, N. and Richardson, J. (2006) 'Parent-training/education programmes in the management of children with conduct disorders', *Journal of Children's Services*, 1: 47–60.

Gould, N., Huxley, P. and Tew, J. (2007) 'Finding a direction for social research in mental health: establishing priorities and developing capacity', *Journal of Social Work*, 7: 177–194.

Gove, W. (1972) 'The relationship between sex roles, marital status and mental health', *Social Forces*, 51: 33–44.

Grant, A., Mills, J., Mulhern, R. and Short, N. (2004) *Cognitive Behavioural Therapy in Mental Health Care*, London: Sage Publications.

Green, H., McGinnity, A., Meltzer, M., Ford, T. and Goodman, R. (2004) *Mental Health of Children and Young People in Great Britain: a survey carried out by the Office of National Statistics for the Department of Health and Scottish executive*, London: Office of National Statistics.

Green, R. (2002) *Mentally Ill Parents and Children's Welfare*. National Society for the Prevention of Cruelty to Children. Online: http://www.nspcc.org.uk/Inform/research/Briefings/mentallyillparents_wda48216.html (accessed 5 May 2009).

Greenberg, M. and Speltz, M. (1993) 'The role of attachment in the early development of disruptive behaviour problems', *Development and Psychopathology*, 5: 191–213.

Harrington, R. (2001) 'Depression, suicide and deliberate self-harm in adolescence', *British Medical Bulletin*, 57: 47–60.

Harris, E.C. and Barraclough, B. (1997) 'Suicide as an outcome for mental disorders: a meta-analysis' *British Journal of Psychiatry*, 170: 205–228.

Harris, N., Williams, S. and Bradshaw, T. (eds) (2002) *Psychosocial Interventions for People with Schizophrenia*, Basingstoke: Palgrave Macmillan.

Harrison, G., Owens, D., Holton, A., Neilson, D. and Boot, D. (1988) 'A prospective study of severe mental disorder in Afro-Caribbean patients', *Psychological Medicine*, 18: 643–657.

Hausman, B. and Hammen, C. (1993) 'Parenting in homeless families: the double crisis', *American Journal of Orthopsychiatry*, 63: 358–369.

Henderson, D. (1939) *Psychopathic States*, New York: Henderson and Co.

Hills, D., LeGrand, J. and Piachaud, D. (eds) (2002) *Understanding Social Exclusion*, Oxford: Oxford University Press.

Hjern, A., Wicks, S. and Dalman, C. (2004) 'Social adversity contributes to high morbidity in psychoses in immigrants: a national cohort study in two generations of Swedish residents', *Psychological Medicine*, 34: 1025–1033.

Hope, R. (2004) *The Ten Essential Shared Capabilities: a framework for the whole of the mental health workforce*, London: Department of Health/National Institute for Mental Health England.

Howarth, C., Kenway, P., Palmer, G. and Street, C. (1998) *Monitoring Poverty and Social Exclusion: Labour's inheritance*, York: Joseph Rowntree Foundation.

Hugman, R. (1991) *Power in Caring Professions*, Basingstoke: Macmillan.

Huxley, P. (2001) 'Editorial: the contribution of social science to mental health services research and development: a SWOT analysis', *Journal of Mental Health*, 10: 117–120.

Huxley, P. (2002) 'Evidence in social care: the policy context', in S. Priebe and M. Slade (eds) *Evidence In Mental Health Care*, Hove: Brunner-Routledge.

Huxley P., Evans, S., Gately, C. and Webber M. (2003) 'Workload and working patterns of mental health social workers: an investigation into occupational pressures – final project report to the Department of Health', London: Institute of Psychiatry.

Huxley, P., Korer, J. and Tolley, S. (1987) 'The psychiatric "caseness" of clients referred to an urban social services department', *British Journal of Social Work*, 17: 507–520.

Institute of Alcohol Studies (2003) *Factsheet: Alcohol and Mental Health*, St Ives: Institute of Alcohol Studies.

Jackson, L. (2002) *Freaks, Geeks and Asperger Syndrome: a user guide to adolescence*, London: Jessica Kingsley.

Jenkins, R., Meltzer, H., Jones, P., Brugha, T., Bebbington, P., Farrell. M., Crepaz-Keay. D. and Knapp, M. (2008) *Foresight Mental Capital and Wellbeing Project. Mental health: future challenges*, London: Government Office for Science.

Jolley, D., Kosky, N. and Holloway, F. (2002) *Caring for People who enter Old Age with Enduring or Relapsing Mental Illness ('Graduates')*, Council Report CR110, London: Royal College of Psychiatrists.

Jolley, D., Kosky, N. and Holloway, F, (2004) 'Older people with long-standing mental illness: the graduates', *Advances in Psychiatric Treatment*, 10: 27–36.

Jones, R. (2008) *Mental Health Act Manual*, 11th edn, London: Sweet and Maxwell.

Kanner, L. (1943) 'Autistic disturbances of affective contact', *Nervous Child*, 2: 217–250.

Jordan, B. and Jordan, C. (2000) *Social Work and the Third Way: tough love as social policy*, London: Sage Publications.

Kendler, K., Thornton, L. and Gardner, C. (2000) 'Stressful life events and previous episodes in the aetiology of major depression in women: an evaluation of the "kindling" hypothesis', *American Journal of Psychiatry*, 157: 1243–1251.

Kendler, K., Thornton, L. and Gardner, C. (2001) 'Genetic risk, number of previous depressive episodes, and stressful life events in predicting onset of major depression', *American Journal of Psychiatry*, 158: 582–586.

Kendler, K., Gardner, C., Neale, M. and Prescott, C. (2001) 'Genetic risk factors for major depression in men and women: similar or different heritabilities and same or partly distinct genes?' *Psychological Medicine*, 31: 605–616.

Kennedy, N., Boydell, J., van Os, J. and Murray, R. (2004) 'Ethnic differences in first clinical presentation of bipolar disorder: results from an epidemiological study', *Journal of Affective Disorders*, 83: 161–168.

King, M. and McKeown, E. (2003) *The Mental Health and Social Wellbeing of Gay Men, Lesbians and Bisexuals in England and Wales*, London: MIND.

King, M., Semlyen, J., See Tai, S., Killaspy, H. Osborn, D., Popelyuk, D. and Nazareth, I. (2008) *Mental Disorders, Suicide and Deliberate Self Harm in Lesbian, Gay and Bisexual People: a systematic review*, London: Care Services Improvement Partnership (CSIP).

King, M., McKeown, E., Warner, J., Ramsay, A., Johnson, K., Cort, C., Wright, L., Blizard, R. and Davidson, O. (2003) 'Mental health and quality of life of gay men and lesbians in England and Wales', *British Journal of Psychiatry*, 183: 552–558.

Kirk, S. and Reid, W. (2002) *Science and Social Work: a critical appraisal*, New York: Columbia University Press.

Kirsch, I. (2000) 'Are drug and placebo effects in depression additive?', *Biological Psychiatry*, 47: 733–735.

Kitwood, T. (1997) *Dementia Reconsidered: the person comes first*, Buckingham: Open University Press.

Kitwood, T. and Benson, S. (eds) (1995) *The New Culture of Dementia Care*, London: Hawker.

Kupfer, D.J. (1991). 'Long-term treatment of depression', *Journal of Clinical Psychiatry*, 52, Suppl. 5: 28–34.

Laing, R.D. (1965) *The Divided Self*, Harmondsworth: Penguin.

Layard, R. (2005) 'Mental illness is now our biggest social problem', speech to the Sainsbury Centre, 14 September 2005. Online: http://www.guardian.co.uk/society/2005/sep/14/mentalhealth.socialcare1 (accessed 4 May 2009).

Leadbeater, C., Bartlett, J. and Gallagher, N. (2008) *Making It Personal*, London: Demos.

Leff, J.P., Kuipers, L., Berkowitz, R., Eberlein-Vries, R. and Sturgeon, D. (1982) 'A controlled trial of social interventions in the families of schizophrenic patients', *British Journal of Psychiatry*, 141: 121–134.

Lehman, A., Myers, C. and Corty, E. (1989) 'Classification of patients with psychiatric and substance abuse syndromes', *Hospital and Community Psychiatry*, 40: 1019–1025.

Lenoir, R. (1974) *Les Exclus*, Paris: Editions de Seuil.

Lewis, G. and Sloggett, A. (1998) 'Suicide, deprivation and unemployment: record linkage study', *British Medical Journal*, 317: 1283–1286.

Lexchin, J., Bero, L.A., Djulbegovic, B. and Clark, O. (2003) 'Pharmaceutical industry sponsorship and research outcome and quality: systematic review', *British Medical Journal*, 326: 1167–1170.

Liabo, K. and Richardson, J. (2007) *Conduct Disorder and Offending Behaviour in Young People: findings from research*, London: Jessica Kingsley.

Lieberman, J.A., Stroup, S., McEvoy, J., Swartz, M., Rosenheck, R., Perkins, D. et al. (2005) 'Clinical Antipsychotic Trials of Intervention Effectiveness (CATIE) investigators. Effectiveness of antipsychotic drugs in patients with chronic schizophrenia', *New England Journal of Medicine*, 353: 1209–1223.

Littlewood, R. and Lipsedge, M. (1997) *Aliens and Alienists: ethnic minorities and psychiatry*, 3rd edn, London: Routledge.

Lloyd, T., Kennedy, N., Fearon, P., Kirkbride, J., Mallett, R., Leff, J. et al. (2005) 'Incidence of bipolar affective disorder in three UK cities: results from the AESOP study', *British Journal of Psychiatry*, 186: 126–131.

Loebel, A.D., Lieberman, J.A., Alvir, J.M., Mayerhoff, D., Geisler, S. and Szymanski, S. (1992) 'Duration of psychosis and outcome in first-episode schizophrenia', *American Journal of Psychiatry*, 149: 1183–1188.

Luntz, B. and Widom, C. (1994) 'Antisocial personality disorder in abused and neglected children', *American Journal of Psychiatry*, 151: 670–674.

Malmberg, L. and Fenton, M. (2001) 'Individual psychodynamic psychotherapy and psychoanalysis for schizophrenia and severe mental illness (Cochrane Review)', *Cochrane Library, Issue 4*, Oxford: Update Software.

Mari, J. and Streiner, D. (1999) 'Family intervention for schizophrenia (Cochrane Review)', *Cochrane Library, Issue 1*, Oxford: Update Software.

Marshall, J. and Watt, P. (1999) *Child Behaviour Problems: a literature review of the size and nature of the problem and prevention interventions in childhood*, Perth, WA: Interagency Committee on Children's Futures.

Marshall, M. (2002) 'Randomised controlled trials: Misunderstanding, fraud and spin', in S. Priebe and M. Slade (eds) *Evidence in Mental Health Care*, Hove: Brunner Routledge.

Maughan, B. and Rutter, M. (1998) 'Continuities and discontinuities in antisocial behaviour from childhood to adult life', *Advances in Clinical Child Psychology*, 20: 1–47.

McCreadie, R. and Kelly, C. (2002) 'Patients with schizophrenia who smoke: private disaster, public resource', *British Journal of Psychiatry*, 176: 109.

McGorry, P.D., Edwards, J., Mihalopoulos, C., Harrigan, S. and Jackson, H. (1996) 'EPPIC: An evolving system of early detection and optimal management', *Schizophrenia Bulletin*, 22: 305–326.

McGuffin, P., Rijsdijk, F., Andrew, M., Sham, P., Katz, R. and Cardno, A. (2003) 'The heritability of bipolar affective disorder and the genetic relationship to unipolar depression', *Archives of General Psychiatry*, 60: 497–502.

McIntosh, A., Cohen, A., Turnbull, N., Esmonde, L, Dennis, P., Eatock, J. et al. (2004) *Clinical Guidelines and Evidence Review for Panic Disorder and Generalised Anxiety Disorder*, Sheffield: University of Sheffield/London: National Collaborating Centre for Primary Care.

McKeith, I. and Fairbairn, A. (2001) 'Biomedical and clinical perspectives', in C. Cantley (ed.) *A Handbook of Dementia Care*, Buckingham: Open University Press.

McKeith, I., Dickson, D., Lowe, J., Emre, M., O'Brien, J.T., Feldman, H. et al. (2005) 'Diagnosis and management of dementia with Lewy Bodies: third report of the DLB consortium', *Neurology*, 65: 1863–1872.

McNeill, A. (2001) *Smoking and Mental Health – A Review of the Literature*, London: Smoke Free London Programme.

Medical Research Council (2001) 'Pathological correlates of late-onset dementia in a multicentre community-based population in England and Wales', *The Lancet*, 357: 169–175.

Meltzer, H., Gill, B., Petticrew, M. and Hinds, K. (1995) *The Prevalence of Psychiatric Morbidity Among Adults Living in Private Households*. OPCS Surveys of Psychiatric Morbidity, Report 1, London: HMSO.

Meltzer, H., Gatward, R. with Goodman, R. and Ford, T. (2000) The *Mental Health of Children and Adolescents in Great Britain. The report of a survey carried out in 1999 by Social Survey Division of the Office for National Statistics on behalf of the Department of Health, the Scottish Health Executive and the National Assembly for Wales*, London: The Stationery Office.

Meltzer, H., Singleton, N., Lee, A., Bebbington, P., Brugha, T. and Jenkins, R. (2002) *The Social and Economic Circumstances of Adults with Mental Disorders*, London: The Stationery Office.

Mental Health Act Commission (2008) *Key Findings about the Use of the Mental Health Act: taken from the Commission's twelfth biannual report 2005–7, risks, rights, recovery*, London: The Stationery Office.

Miller, P. and Rose, N. (eds) (1986) *The Power of Psychiatry*, Cambridge: Polity.

Mills, J., Mulhern, R., Grant, A. and Short, N. (2004) 'Working with people who have complex emotional and relationship difficulties (borderlines or people?)' in A. Grant, J. Mills, R. Mulhern and N. Short (eds) *Cognitive Behavioural Therapy in Mental Health Care*, London: Sage Publications.

Moran, P., Jenkins, R., Tylee, A., Blizard, R. and Mann, A. (2000) 'The prevalence of personality disorder among UK primary care attenders', *Acta Psychiatrica Scandinavica*, 102: 52–57.

Morgan, C., Burns, T., Fitzpatrick, R., Pinfold, V. and Priebe, S. (2007) 'Social exclusion and mental health: conceptual and methodological review', *British Journal of Psychiatry*, 191: 477–483.

Mowlam, A. and Lewis, J. (2005) *Exploring How General Practitioners Work with Patients on Sick Leave*, DWP Research Report 257, Corporate Document Services, London: Department of Work and Pensions.

Mulhern, M., Short, N., Grant, A. and Mills, M. (2004) 'Working with people who are depressed', in A. Grant, J. Mills, R. Mulhern and N. Short (eds) *Cognitive Behavioural Therapy in Mental Health Care*, London: Sage Publications.

Murray, L. (1996) 'Personal and social influences on parenting and adult adjustment' in S. Kraemer and J. Roberts (eds) *The Politics of Attachment: towards a secure society*, London: Free Association Books.

National Audit Office (2007) *Improving Services and Support for People with Dementia,* London: The Stationery Office.

National Collaborating Centre for Mental Health (2003) *Schizophrenia. Full national clinical guideline on core interventions for primary and secondary care,* London: The British Psychological Society and Gaskell.

National Collaborating Centre for Mental Health (2004) *Depression: management of depression in primary and secondary care,* London: British Psychological Society and Gaskell.

National Collaborating Centre for Mental Health (2005a) *Depression in Children and Young People: identification and management in primary, community and secondary care,* London: British Psychological Society and Gaskell.

National Collaborating Centre for Mental Health (2005b) *Post-traumatic Stress Disorder: the management of PTSD in primary and secondary care,* London: British Psychological Society and Gaskell.

National Collaborating Centre for Mental Health (2006a) *A NICE-SCIE Guideline on Supporting People with Dementia and their Carers in Health and Social Care, National Clinical Practice Guideline Number 42,* London: The British Psychological Society and Gaskell.

National Collaborating Centre for Mental Health (2006b) *The Management of Bipolar Disorder in Adults, Children and Young People, in Primary and Secondary Care,* London: The British Psychological Society and Gaskell.

National Collaborating Centre for Mental Health (2008) *Attention Deficit Hyperactiviy Disorder: diagnosis and management of children, young people and adults. National Clinical Practice Guideline No. 72,* London: British Psychological Society and Royal College of Psychiatrists.

National Collaborating Centre for Mental Health (2009) *Schizophrenia. Full national clinical guideline on core interventions for primary and secondary care (Update),* London: The British Psychological Society and Gaskell.

National Institute for Clinical Excellence (2003) *Guidance on the Use of Electroconvulsive Therapy, Technology Appraisal No. 59,* London: National Institute for Clinical Excellence.

National Institute for Mental Health England (2003) *Personality Disorder: no longer a diagnosis of exclusion,* London: Department of Health.

Newbigging, K. with Lowe, J. (2005) *Direct Payments and Mental Health: new directions,* York: Joseph Rowntree Foundation.

Newbigging, K., McKeown, M., Hunkins-Hutchinson, E. and French, B. (2007) *Mtetezi: mental health advocacy with African and Caribbean men,* London: Social Care Institute for Excellence.

NICE (2008) *Antisocial Personality Disorder: treatment, management and prevention,* London: National Institute for Health and Clinical Excellence.

Office for National Statistics (2003) *Labour Force Survey,* August. Online: http://www.statistics.gov.uk/downloads/theme_labour/lfsqs_0803.pdf (accessed 7 May 2009).

Office of the Deputy Prime Minister (2004) *Mental Health and Social Exclusion: social exclusion unit report,* London: Office of the Deputy Prime Minister.

O'Leary, P. and Gould, N. (2008) 'Men who were sexually abused in childhood and subsequent suicidal ideation: community comparison, explanations and practice implications', *British Journal of Social Work.* Advanced access published 1 October, doi:10.1093/bjsw/bcn130.

Oliver, M. and Barnes, C. (1998) *Disability and Social Policy: from exclusion to inclusion,* Harlow: Adison Wesley Longman.

Onyett, S. (2003) *Teamworking in Mental Health,* Basingstoke: Palgrave Macmillan.

Osher, F. and Kofoed, L. (1989) 'Treatments of patients with psychiatric and psychoactive substance abuse disorders', *Hospital and Community Psychiatry,* 40: 1025–1030.

Paris, J. (2003) *Personality Disorders over Time: precursors, course, and outcome.* Arlington, VA: American Psychiatric Publishing.

Parr, H., Philo, C. and Burns, N. (2004) 'Social geographies of rural mental health: experiencing inclusions and exclusions', *Transactions of the Institute of British Geographers*, 29: 401–419.

Paton, J., Johnston, K., Katona, C. and Livingston, G. (2004) 'What causes problems in Alzheimers disease: attributions by caregivers. A qualitative study', *International Journal of Geriatric Psychiatry*, 19: 527–532.

Pawson, R., Boaz, A., Grayson, L., Long, A. and Barnes, C. (2003) *Types and Quality of Knowledge in Social Care: Knowledge Review 3*, London, Social Care Institute for Excellence.

Payne, M. (2005) *Modern Social Work Theory*, 3rd edn, Basingstoke: Palgrave Macmillan.

Payne, M. and Reith, M. (2009) *Social Work in End-of-Life and Palliative Care*, Bristol: Policy Press.

Payne, S. (2006) 'Mental health poverty and social exclusion', in C. Pantazis, D. Gordon, and R. Levitas (eds) *Poverty and Social Exclusion in Britain*, Bristol: Policy Press.

Peck, E., Gulliver, P. and Towell, D. (2002) *Modernising Partnerships: an evaluation of Somerset's Innovations in the Commissioning and Organisation of Mental Health Services*, London: Institute for Applied Health and Social Policy.

Phelan, M., Stradins, L. and Morrison, S. (2001) 'Physical health of people with severe mental illness', *British Journal of Psychiatry*, 322: 443–444.

Phillipson, C. (1982) *Capitalism and the Construction of Old Age*, London: Macmillan.

Pilgrim, D. (2002) 'The biopsychosocial model in Anglo-American psychiatry: past present and future?', *Journal of Mental Health*, 11: 585–594.

Pilling, S., Bebbington, P., Kuipers, E., Garety, G., Geddes, J., Martindale, B., Orbach, G. and Morgan, C. (2002) 'Psychological treatments in schizophrenia: I. Meta-analysis of family intervention and cognitive behaviour therapy', *Psychological Medicine*, 32: 763–782.

Plumpton, M. and Bostock, J. (2003) *Income, Poverty and Mental Health: a literature review*, Newcastle: Department of Psychological Services and Research, North Tyneside and Northumberland NHS Mental Health Trust.

Porter, R. (2003) *Madness: a brief history*, Oxford: Oxford University Press.

Prins, H. (1980) *Offenders, Deviants or Patients? An introduction to the study of socio-forensic problems*, London: Tavistock Publications.

Prins, H. (1999) *Will They Do It Again? Risk assessment and management in criminal justice and society*, London: Routledge.

Prior, M., Smart, D., Sanson, A. and Oberklaid, F. (1993) 'Sex differences in psychological adjustment from infancy to 8 years', *Journal of the American Academy of Child and Adolescent Psychiatry*, 32: 291–305.

Pritchard, C. (2006) *Mental Health Social Work: evidence-based practice*, London: Routledge.

Pritchard, R. (2006) 'The accommodation dimension: housing and mental disorder', in C. Pritchard (ed.), *Mental Health Social Work: evidence-based practice*, London: Routledge.

Prochaska, J. and DiClemente, C. (1986) 'Towards a comprehensive model of change', in L. Miller and N. Heather (eds) *Treating Addictive Behaviours: process of change*, New York: Plenum.

Pugh, R. and Gould, N. (2000) 'Globalization, social work and social welfare', *European Journal of Social Work*, 3: 123–138.

Putnam, R. (2000) *Bowling Alone: the collapse and revival of American community*, New York: Simon and Schuster.

Rack, P. (1982) *Race, Culture and Mental Disorder*, London: Tavistock.

Rai-Atkins, A., Ali Jama, A., Wright, N., Scott, V., Perring, C., Craig, G. and Katbamna, S. (2002) *Best Practice in Mental Health; advocacy for African, Caribbean and South Asian communities*, York: Joseph Rowntree Foundation.

Raleigh, V. and Balarajan, R. (1992) 'Suicide and self-burning among Indians and West Indians in England and Wales', *British Journal of Psychiatry*, 129: 365–368.

Ralph, R. and Corrigan, P. (eds) (2005) *Recovery in Mental Illness: broadening our understanding of wellness*, Washington DC: American Psychological Association.

Ramchandani, P. and Stein. A. (2003) 'The impact of parental psychiatric disorder on children', *British Medical Journal*, 327: 242–243.

Rapp, C. and Wintersteen, R. (1989) 'The strengths model of case management', *Psychosocial Rehabilitation Journal*, 13: 23–32.

Redmond, B. (2005) 'Homelessness and mental health' in S. Quin and B. Redmond (eds) *Mental Health and Social Policy in Ireland*, Dublin: University College Dublin.

Reid, W. (1978) *The Task-Centered System*, New York: Columbia University Press.

Reid, W. and Epstein, L. (1972) *Task-Centered Casework*, New York: Columbia University Press.

Reid, W. and Shyne, A. (1969) *Brief and Extended Casework*, New York: Columbia University Press.

Rethink (2008) *Briefing – physical health and mental health*. Online: http://www.rethink.org/how_we_can_help/news_and_media/briefing_notes/briefing_5.html (accessed 14 January 2009).

Rhodes, M. (1986) *Ethical Dilemmas in Social Work Practice*, Boston, MA: Routledge.

Richardson, J. and Joughin, C. (2002) *Parent-Training Programmes for the Management of Young Children with Conduct Disorders: findings from research*, London: Gaskell.

Riddell, S., Pearson, C., Jolly, D., Barnes, C. Priestley, M. and Mercer, G. (2005) 'The development of direct payments in the UK: implications for social justice', *Social Policy and Society*, 4: 75–85.

Ridgeway, S. (1997) 'Deaf people and psychological health – some preliminary findings', *Deaf Worlds*, 1: 9–17.

Ridley, J. and Jones, L. (2003) 'Direct what? The untapped potential of direct payments to users of mental health services', *Disability and Society*, 18: 643–658.

Ritchie, J., Dick D. and Lingham, R. (1994) *The Report of the Inquiry into the Care and Treatment of Christopher Clunis*, London: HMSO.

Roberts, G. and Wolfson, P. (2006) 'New directions in rehabilitation: learning from the recovery movement', in G. Roberts, S. Davenport, F. Holloway and T. Tattan (eds) *Enabling Recovery: the principles and practice of rehabilitation psychiatry*, London: Gaskell.

Robins, L. (1991) 'Conduct disorder', *Journal of Child Psychology and Psychiatry*, 32: 193–212.

Robjant, K., Hassan, R. and Katona, C. (2009) 'Mental health implications of detaining asylum seekers', *British Journal of Psychiatry*, 194: 306–312.

Rogers, A. and Pilgrim, D. (2001) *Mental Health Policy in Britain*, 2nd edn, Basingstoke: Palgrave.

Rogers, A. and Pilgrim, D. (2003) *Mental Health and Inequality*, Basingstoke: Palgrave Macmillan.

Rogers, P. and Curran, C. (2004) 'Working with people in forensic settings' in A. Grant, J. Mills, R. Mulhern and N. Short (eds) *Cognitive Behavioural Therapy in Mental Health Care*, London: Sage Publications.

Rose, D. (ed.) (2001) *Users Voices*, London: Sainsbury Centre for Mental Health.

Rose, D., Fleischmann, P., Wykes, T. Leese, M. and Bindman, J. (2003) 'Patients' perspectives on electroconvulsivetherapy: systematic review', *British Medical Journal*, 326: 1343–1344.

Rose, N. (2007) 'Psychopharmaceuticals in Europe', in M. Knapp, D. McDaid, E. Mossialos and G. Thornicroft (eds) *Mental Health Policy and Practice Across Europe*, Maidenhead: Open University Press.

Rose, S., Bisson, J. and Wessely, S. (2004) 'Psychological debriefing for preventing post traumatic stress disorder (PTSD) (Cochrane review)', *Cochrane Library, Issue 3*, Chichester: John Wiley.

Ross, R., Fabiano, E. and Ewles, C. (1988) 'Reasoning and rehabilitation', *International Journal of Offender Therapy and Comparative Criminology*, 32: 29–35.

Royal College of Psychiatry (2009) *Physical Health in Mental Health: final report of a scoping group, Occasional paper 67*, London: Royal College of Psychiatrists.

Ruch, G. (2005) 'Relationship-based and reflective practice in contemporary child care social work', *Child and Family Social Work*, 4: 111–124.

Rutter, M. (1989) 'Psychiatric disorder in parents as a risk factor for children' in D. Schaffer (ed.) *Prevention of Mental Disorder, Alcohol* and *Other Drug Use in Children and Adolescents*, Rockville, MD: Office for Substance Abuse, USDHHS.

Rutter, M. (2003) 'Poverty and child mental health', *JAMA*, 290: 2063–2064.

Rutter, M. and Giller, H. (1983) *Juvenile Delinquency Trends and Perspectives*, New York: Penguin Books.

Rutter, M. and Quinton, D. (1984) 'Parental psychiatric disorder: effects on children', *Psychological Medicine*, 14: 853–880.

Sainsbury Centre for Mental Health (2001) *The Capable Practitioner Framework: a framework and list of the practitioner capabilities required to implement the National Service Framework for Mental Health*, London: Sainsbury Centre for Mental Health.

Sainsbury Centre for Mental Health, (2002) *Breaking the Circles of Fear: a review of the relationship between mental health services and African and Caribbean communities*, London: Sainsbury Centre for Mental Health.

Sainsbury Centre for Mental Health (2003) *The Economic and Social Costs of Mental Illness*, London: Sainsbury Centre for Mental Health.

Sainsbury Centre for Mental Health (2006) *First Steps to Work – a study at Broadmoor Hospital. Briefing 30*, London: Sainsbury Centre for Mental Health.

Sainsbury Centre for Mental Health (2007) 'Anti social behaviour orders and mental health: the evidence to date'. Online: http://www.scmh.org.uk/pdfs/asbo_consultation_response_nov07.pdf (accessed 8 May 2009).

Sartorius, N. (2001) 'The economic and social burden of depression', *Journal of Clinical Psychiatry*, 62 (Suppl 15): 8–11.

Sashidharan, S. (2001) 'Institutional racism in British psychiatry', *Psychiatric Bulletin*, 25: 244–247.

Sayce, L. and Curran, C. (2007) 'Tackling social exclusion across Europe', in M. Knapp, D. McDaid, E. Mossialos and G. Thornicroft (eds) *Mental Health Policy and Practice Across Europe*, Maidenhead: Open University Press.

Schneider, J. (1993) 'Care programming in mental health: assimilation and adaptation', *British Journal of Social Work*, 23: 383–403.

Schneider, K. (1923) *Die Psychopathischen Personlichkeiten*, Berlin: Springer.

Schneider, K. (1959) *Clinical Psychopathology*, 5th edn, New York: Grune and Stratton.

Scull, A. (1977) *Decarceration: community treatment and the deviant*, Cambridge: Polity.

Sedgwick, P. (1972) 'R.D. Laing: self, symptom and society', in R. Boyers and R. Orrill (eds) *Laing and Anti-Psychiatry*, Harmondsworth: Penguin Education.

Sedgwick, P. (1982) *Psycho Politics*, London: Pluto.

Shah, P. and Mountain, D. (2007) 'The medical model is dead – long live the medical model', *British Journal of Psychiatry*, 191: 375–377.

Shaikh, S. (1985) 'Cross-cultural comparison, psychiatric admission of Asian and indigenous patients in Leicestershire', *International Journal of Social Psychiatry*, 31: 3–11.

Shega, J., Levin, A., Hougham, G., Cox Haley, D., Luchins, D., Hanrahan, P. et al. (2003) 'Palliative Excellence in Alzheimer Care Efforts (PEACE): a program description', *Journal of Palliative Medicine*, 6: 315–320.

Sheppard, M. (1993) 'Maternal depression and child care: the significance for social work and social work research', *Adoption and Fostering*, 17: 10–15.

Sheppard, M. (2001) 'Depressed mothers' experience of partnership in child and family care', *British Journal of Social Work*, 32: 93–112.

Showalter, E. (1987) *The Female Malady: women, madness and English culture*, London: Virago.

Shulman, K. (1993) 'Mania in the elderly', *International Review of Psychiatry*, 5: 445–453.

Singh, S. and Burns, T. (2006) 'Race and mental health: there is more to race than racism', *British Medical Journal*, 333: 648–651.

Singleton, N., Bumpstead, R., O'Brien, M., Lee, A. and Meltzer, H. (2001) *Psychiatric Morbidity Among Adults Living in Private Households, 2000*, London: The Stationery Office.

Skills for Care (2008) *Developing Skills: leadership and management*. Online: http://www.skillsforcare.org.uk/developing_skills/leadership_and_management/leadership_and_management_introduction.aspx (accessed 9 May 2009).

Smith, A. and Twomey, B. (2002) 'Labour market experiences of people with disabilities', *Labour Market Trends*, August: 415–427.

Social Care Institute for Excellence (2007a) *Understanding Later Stage Dementia*, London: Social Care Institute for Excellence. Online: http://www.scie.org.uk/publications/elearning/mentalhealth/mh06/index.asp (accessed 7 May 2009).

Social Care Institute for Excellence (2007b) *Common Mental Health Problems Among Older People*, London: Social Care Institute for Excellence. Online: http://www.scie.org.uk/publications/elearning/mentalhealth/mh04/resource/html/object4/index.htm (accessed 7 May 2009).

Social Perspectives Network (2004) *Integration of Health and Social Care: promoting social care perspectives within integrated mental health services*, London: Social Perspectives Network.

Sorensen, S., Pinquart, M. and Duberstein, P. (2002) 'How effective are interventions with caregivers? An updated meta-analysis', *The Gerontologist*, 42: 356–372.

STAKES (1999) *Introduction to Mental Health Issues in the EU*, Helsinki: Finnish Ministry of Social Affairs and Health.

Stonewall (2008) *Frequently Asked Questions.* Online: http://www.stonewall.org.uk/information_bank/frequently_asked_questions/default.asp (accessed 3 June 2008).

Sullivan, G., Burnham, A. and Koegel, P. (2000) 'Pathways to homelessness amongst the mentally ill', *Social Psychiatry and Psychiatric Epidemiology*, 35: 444–450.

Szasz, T. (1971) *The Manufacture of Madness*, London: Routledge and Kegan Paul.

Tanenbaum, S. (2003) 'Evidence-based practice in mental health: practical weaknesses meet political strengths', *Journal of Evaluation in Clinical Practice*, 2: 287–301.

Tanner, D. and Harris, J. (2008) *Working with Older People*, London: Routledge.

Targosz, S., Bebbington, P., Lewis, G., Brugha, T., Jenkins, R., Farrell, M. and Melzer, H. (2003) 'Lone mothers, social exclusion and depression', *Psychological Medicine*, 33: 715–722.

Tarpey, M. and Watson, L. (1997) *Housing Need in Merton: people with severe mental illness living in households*, London: London Borough of Merton.

Taylor, P. and Gunn, J (1999) 'Homicides by people with mental illness: myth and reality', *British Journal of Psychiatry*, 174: 9–14.

Tew, J. (2002) 'Going social: championing a holistic model of mental distress within professional education', *Social Work Education*, 1: 143–156.

Tew, J., Gould, N., Abankwa, D., Barnes, H., Beresford, P., Carr, S. et al. (2006) *Values and Methodologies For Social Research in Mental Health*, Bristol: Policy Press.

Thompson, N. (2000) *Understanding Social Work: Preparing For Practice*, London: Macmillan.

Thornicroft, G. and Tansella, M. (2004) 'Components of a modern mental health service: a pragmatic balance of community and hospital care', *British Journal of Psychiatry*, 185: 283–290.

Truax, C. and Carkhuff, R. (1967) *Towards Effective Counseling and Psychotherapy Training and Practice*, Chicago: Aldine Atherton.

Tucker (1999) *Treatment of Survivors of Motor Vehicle Accidents*, 2nd edn, Washington, DC: APA.

Tunnard, R. (2004) *Parental Mental Health Problems: key messages from research, policy and practice*, Dartington: Research In Practice.

Wallcraft, J. and Bryant, M. (2003) *The Mental Health Service User Movement in England*, London: Sainsbury Centre for Mental Health.

Walsh, C.L., Gordon, M.F., Marshall. M., Wilson, F. and Hunt, T. (2005) 'Interprofessional capability: a developing framework for inter-professional education', *Nurse Education in Practice*, 5: 230–237.

Warner, J., McKeown, E., Griffin, M., Johnson, K., Ramsay, A. and King, M. (2004) 'Rates and predictors of mental illness in gay men, lesbians and bisexual men and women', *British Journal of Psychiatry*, 185: 479–485.

Webb, D. and Harris R. (eds) (1999) *Mentally Disordered Offenders: managing people nobody owns*, London: Routledge.

Webb, S. (2006) *Social Work in a Risk Society: social and political perspectives*, Basingstoke: Palgrave Macmillan.

Webber, M. (2005) 'Social capital and mental health', in J. Tew (ed.) *Social Perspectives in Mental Health*, London: Jessica Kingsley.

Webber, M. (2008) *Evidence-based Policy and Practice in Mental Health Social Work*, Exeter: Learning Matters.

Webber, M. and Huxley, P. (2004) 'Social exclusion and risk of emergency compulsory and admission', *Social Psychiatry and Psychiatric Epidemiology*, 39: 1000–1009.

Weich, S. and Lewis, G. (1998) 'Poverty, unemployment and common mental disorders: population based cohort study', *British Medical Journal*, 317: 115–119.

Weich, S., Lewis, G. and Jenkins, S. (2001) 'Income inequality and the prevalence of common mental disorders in Britain', *British Journal of Psychiatry*, 178: 22–27.

Wells, R., Jinnett, K., Alexander, J., Lichtenstein, R., Liu, D. and Zazzali, J. (2006) 'Team leadership and patient outcomes in US psychiatric treatment settings', *Social Science and Medicine*, 62: 1840–1852.

White, S. (1996) 'Regulating mental health and motherhood in contemporary welfare services: anxious attachment or attachment anxiety?', *Critical Social Policy*, 16: 67–94.

Whitley, E., Gunnell, D., Dorling, D. and Smith, G. (1999) 'Ecological study of social fragmentation, poverty and suicide', *British Medical Journal*, 319: 1034–1037.

Wilkinson, R. (2001) 'Social status, inequality and health', in T. Heller, R. Muston, M. Sidell and C. Lloyd (eds) *Working for Health*, London: Open University Press and Sage Publications.

Williams, C. (2003) *From Social Care to Social Inclusion*, York: Northern Centre for Mental Health.

Williams, R. and Avebury, K. (1995) *A Place in Mind: commissioning and providing mental health services for people who are homeless*, London: HMSO.

Williams, S. (2002) 'The nature of schizophrenia', in N. Harris, S. Williams and T. Bradshaw, (eds) *Psychosocial Interventions for People with Schizophrenia*, Basingstoke: Palgrave Macmillan.

Wilson, K., Ruch, G., Lymbery, M. and Cooper, A. (2008) *Social Work: an introduction to contemporary practice*, Harlow: Pearson Longman.

Wright, S., Gournay, K., Glorney, F. and Thornicroft, G. (2000) 'Dual diagnosis in the suburbs: prevalence, need and inpatient service use', *Social Psychiatry and Psychiatric Epidemiology*, 35: 297–304.

World Health Organization (1992) *International Classification of Diseases and Health Related Problems*, Geneva: World Health Organization.

World Health Organization (2002) *Word Health Report 2002*, Geneva: World Health Organization.

Zwarenstein, M., Reeves, S., Barr, H., Hammick, M., Koppel, I. and Atkins, J. (2002) *Interprofessional Education: effects on professional practice and health care outcomes (Cochrane review), issue 4*, London: The Cochrane Library.

Index

7550